INTRAVENOUS MEDICATIONS FOR
CRITICAL

SECOND EDITION

Robert M. Lester, M.D., F.A.C.C.

Director, Coronary Care Unit
Graduate Hospital
Associate Clinical Professor
University of Pennsylvania
Philadelphia, Pennsylvania

Ann Marie Dente-Cassidy, R.N., M.S.N.

Clinical Editor
Critical Care Educator
Spring City, Pennsylvania

Reviewed by: Susan S. Lester, B.S. Pharmacy, Philadelphia, Pennsylvania
Acknowledgement: Veronica Mitchell, Department of Anesthesia, Johns Hopkins Hospital, Baltimore, Maryland

W.B. SAUNDERS COMPANY
A Division of Harcourt Brace & Company

Philadelphia London
Montreal Sydney

W.B. SAUNDERS COMPANY
A Division of Harcourt Brace & Company

The Curtis Center
Independence Square West
Philadelphia, Pennsylvania 19106

Library of Congress Cataloging-in-Publication Data

Lester, Robert M.
Intravenous medications for critical care / Robert M. Lester, Ann Marie Dente-Cassidy ; reviewed by Susan S. Lester, Veronica Mitchell.—2nd ed.
p. cm.
Dente-Cassidy's name appeared first on earlier edition.
ISBN 0-7216-4887-8
1. Injections, Intravenous—Handbooks, manuals, etc. 2. Intravenous therapy—Handbooks, manuals, etc. 3. Intensive care nursing—Handbooks, manuals, etc. I. Dente-Cassidy, Ann Marie. II. Title.
[DNLM: 1. Infusions, Intravenous—nurses' instruction—handbooks. 2. Critical Care—nurses' instruction—handbooks. 3. Drugs--administration & dosage—nurses' instruction—handbooks. WB 39 L642i 1995]
RM170.L47 1995 615.5'8—dc20
DNLM/DLC 95-3557

Intravenous Medications for Critical Care ISBN 0–7216–4887–8

Printed in the United States of America Last digit is the print number: 9 8 7 6 5 4 3 2 1

Contents

Sources

American Society of Hospital Pharmacists: Clin Pharmacy 12, 1993.

Emergency Cardiac Care Committee and Subcommittees, American Heart Association: *Advanced Cardiac Life Support Guidelines.* JAMA 268:2199–2241, 1992.

Connor CS, Rumack BH (eds): *Drug Dex.* Micromedix Inc. (Poisindex Co.), (Computer Software) vol. 79, 1994. University of Colorado, Boulder, CO.

Marini JJ, Wheeler AP: *Critical Care Medicine—The Essentials.* Baltimore, Williams & Wilkins, 1989.

Marino PL: *The ICU Book.* Malvern, PA, Lea & Febiger, 1991.

McEvoy GK: *American Hospital Formulary Service.* Bethesda, MD, American Society of Hospital Pharmacists, 1994.

Olon BR (ed): *Facts and Comparisons.* St. Louis, Walters Kluwer, 1993.

Physicians' Desk Reference (P.D.R.). Oradell, NJ, Medical Economics Company, 1994.

Shargel L, Yu AB: *Applied BioPharmaceutics and Pharmacokinetics.* Norwalk, CT, Appleton-Century-Crofts, 1985.

Instruction Card 1

Aminocaproic Acid (Amicar)

15 grams in 250 ml

■ Infusion Rate in mL/hr (pump setting) ■ Drug Dose in g/hr

mL/hr	g/hr	mL/hr	g/hr	mL/hr	g/hr	mL/hr	g/hr	mL/hr	g/hr	mL/hr	g/hr
1	0.06	21	1.26	41	2.46	61	3.66	81	4.86	101	6.06
2	0.12	22	1.32	42	2.52						
3	0.18	23	1.38	43	2.58						
4	0.24	24	1.44	44	2.64						
5	0.30	25	1.50	45	2.70						
6	0.36	26	1.56	46	2.76						
7	0.42	27	1.62	47	2.82						
8	0.48	28	1.68	48	2.88						
9	0.54	29	1.74	49	2.94						
10	0.60	30	1.80	50	3.00						
11	0.66	31	1.86	51	3.06						
12	0.72	32	1.92	52	3.12						
13	0.78	33	1.98	53	3.18						
14	0.84	34	2.04	54	3.24						
15	0.90	35	2.10	55	3.30						
16	0.96	36	2.16	56	3.36						
17	1.02	37	2.22	57	3.42						
18	1.08	38	2.28	58	3.48	78	4.68	98	5.88	118	7.08
19	1.14	39	2.34	59	3.54	79	4.74	99	5.94	119	7.14
20	1.20	40	2.40	60	3.60	80	4.80	100	6.00	120	7.20

To find: amount of drug being delivered

Known: present infusion rate (pump setting)

1. Be sure drug concentration being used matches the concentration shown on table.
2. Locate known infusion rate or pump setting (red number). Infusion rate is given in mL/hour.
3. Follow that red number horizontally across to the drug dosage beside it (black number).

Instruction Cards 2 and 3
Dopamine Hydrochloride (Intropin)

400 mg in 500 mL

DRUG DOSE in μg/kg/min

Patient's Weight

Infusion Rate in mL/hr — kg / lbs	40 / 88	45 / 99	50 / 110	55 / 121	60 / 132	65 / 143	70 / 154	75 / 165	80 / 176	85 / 187	90 / 198	95 / 209	100 / 220	105 / 231	110 / 242
5	1.7	1.5	1.3	1.2	1.1	1.0	1.0								
10	3.3	3.0	2.7	2.4	2.2	2.1	1.9								
15	5.0	4.4	4.0	3.6	3.3	3.1	2.9								
20	6.7	5.9	5.3	4.8	4.4	4.1	3.8								
25	8.3	7.4	6.7	6.1	5.6	5.1	4.8								
30	10.0	8.9	8.0	7.3	6.7	6.2	5.7								
35	11.7	10.4	9.3	8.5	7.8	7.2	6.7								
40	13.3	11.9	10.7	9.7	8.9	8.2	7.6								
45	15.0	13.3	12.0	10.9	10.0	9.2	8.6								
50	16.7	14.8	13.3	12.1	11.1	10.3	9.5								
55	18.3	16.3	14.7	13.3	12.2	11.3	10.5								
60	20.0	17.8	16.0	14.5	13.3	12.3	11.4								
65	21.7	19.3	17.3	15.8	14.4	13.3	12.4								
70	23.3	20.7	18.7	17.0	15.6	14.4	13.3								
75	25.0	22.2	20.0	18.2	16.7	15.4	14.3								
80	26.7	23.7	21.3	19.4	17.8	16.4	15.2								
85	28.3	25.2	22.7	20.6	18.9	17.4	16.2								
90	30.0	26.7	24.0	21.8	20.0	18.5	17.1								
95	31.7	28.1	25.3	23.0	21.1	19.5	18.1								
100	33.3	29.8	26.7	24.2	22.2	20.5	19.0								
105	35.0	31.1	28.0	25.5	23.3	21.5	20.0								
110	36.7	32.6	29.3	26.7	24.4	22.6	21.0								
115	38.3	34.1	30.7	27.9	25.6	23.6	21.9								
120	40.0	35.6	32.0	29.1	26.7	24.6	22.9								

To find: correct infusion rate (pump setting) in mL/hour for the patient's weight and prescribed dose

Known: prescribed drug dosage and patient's weight

1. Be sure drug concentration being used matches the concentration shown on table.
2. Find the patient's weight (to the closest 5 lb or 11 kg) at the top of table.
3. Follow vertically down the appropriate weight column to find the prescribed drug dosage.
4. Follow that number horizontally to the far left column (red number) to locate the corresponding infusion rate (pump setting) given in mL/hour.

DRUG DOSE in µg/kg/min

Infusion Rate in mL/hr	Patient's Weight kg / lbs: 40 / 88	45 / 99	50 / 110	55 / 121	60 / 132	65 / 143	70 / 154	75 / 165	80 / 176	85 / 187	90 / 198	95 / 209	100 / 220	105 / 231	110 / 242
5	1.7	1.5	1.3	1.2	1.1	1.0	1.0								
10	3.3	3.0	2.7	2.4	2.2	2.1	1.9								
15	5.0	4.4	4.0	3.6	3.3	3.1	2.9								
20	6.7	5.9	5.3	4.8	4.4	4.1	3.8								
25	8.3	7.4	6.7	6.1	5.6	5.1	4.8								
30	10.0	8.9	8.0	7.3	6.7	6.2	5.7								
35	11.7	10.4	9.3	8.5	7.8	7.2	6.7								
40	13.3	11.9	10.7	9.7	8.9	8.2	7.6								
45	15.0	13.3	12.0	10.9	10.0	9.2	8.6								
50	16.7	14.8	13.3	12.1	11.1	10.3	9.5								
55	18.3	16.3	14.7	13.3	12.2	11.3	10.5								
60	20.0	17.8	16.0	14.5	13.3	12.3	11.4								
65	21.7	19.3	17.3	15.8	14.4	13.3	12.4								
70	23.3	20.7	18.7	17.0	15.6	14.4	13.3								
75	25.0	22.2	20.0	18.2	16.7	15.4	14.3								
80	26.7	23.7	21.3	19.4	17.8	16.4	15.2								
85	28.3	25.2	22.7	20.6	18.9	17.4	16.2								
90	30.0	26.7	24.0	21.8	20.0	18.5	17.1								
95	31.7	28.1	25.3	23.0	21.1	19.5	18.1								
100	33.3	29.8	26.7	24.2	22.2	20.5	19.0								
105	35.0	31.1	28.0	25.5	23.3	21.5	20.0								
110	36.7	32.6	29.3	26.7	24.4	22.6	21.0								
115	38.3	34.1	30.7	27.9	25.6	23.6	21.9								
120	40.0	35.6	32.0	29.1	26.7	24.6	22.9								

To find: amount of medication being delivered for patient's weight (µg/kg/min)

Known: present infusion rate (pump setting)

1. Be sure drug concentration being used matches the concentration shown on table.
2. Locate the known infusion rate (red number) in the far left column given in mL/hour.
3. Locate the patient's weight (to the closest 5 lb or 11 kg) from top of table.
4. Move vertically down the weight column while moving horizontally across from the infusion rate (pump setting) to where the two intersect. That intersecting number is the amount of medication being delivered (µg/kg/min).

Administrative Guidelines

Completely familiarize yourself with the contents of each drug card before initiating therapy.

■ These cards are not intended for use in pediatric patients because drug safety and efficacy have not, in general, been established.

■ The safety of these medications in pregnant women has not been established, and their use is not recommended unless no alternative therapy is available.

■ Emergency and resuscitative equipment and medications should always be immediately available during drug administration to manage untoward reactions.

■ Decrease dose or terminate infusion if adverse effects are noted or toxicity is suspected.

■ Terminate infusion if precipitate or unusual discoloration is observed.

■ Do not administer any of the infusions in a "piggyback" manner to an existing infusion unless confirmation of compatibility is documented.

■ It is recommended that these medications be piggybacked into an existing open intravenous (IV) line of 5% dextrose and water or 0.9% saline as a safety measure in case of untoward effects.

■ Each of the infusion tables is based on a specific drug dose in a precise volume of diluent. Overfill of intravenous bags and bottles by manufacturers may prevent accurate drug dosing. A more precise infusion dose can be achieved by withdrawing a volume of drug-free fluid from the infusion bottle/bag equal to that added during admixture.

■ The concentrations selected for the infusion tables have been chosen both to be practical and to conform to drug dose guidelines. Alternative concentration infusions may be indicated, for example, when fluid restriction is necessary. It is suggested that a multiple (e.g., 2×, 3×, 4×) of the concentration presented be employed to simplify mathematical calculation of delivered drug dose.

■ These cards are designed to facilitate proper and safe administration of the intravenous infusion drugs. They are not designed to be a definitive reference. In the event that further information is desired, consult the drug manufacturer or published sources.

■ In the event that inadequate clinical response is noted, consider subtherapeutic dosing, inappropriate drug selection, misdiagnosis, or interference by concomitant drugs or clinical conditions.

Drug Calculation Formulae

To Calculate Drug Concentration per mL (cc)

$$\frac{\text{Known amount of drug (D)}}{\text{Total volume of diluent (V)}} = \text{Amount of drug/mL (concentration)}$$

Example: $$\frac{\text{400 mg dopamine}}{\text{500 mL D5W}} = \frac{\text{0.8 mg}}{\text{mL}} \text{ or 800 µg/mL}$$

To Calculate Dose/min with Infusion Rate Given

$$\frac{\text{Concentration (dose)} \times \text{Infusion Rate}}{\text{60 min}} = \text{dose/min}$$

Example: A patient is receiving 30 mL/hr of a dopamine infusion with a concentration of 400 mg dopamine/500 mL D5W (800 µg/mL):

$$\frac{\text{800 µg/mL} \times \text{30 mL/60 min}}{\text{60 min}} = \text{400 µg/min}$$

To Calculate Infusion Rate (IR) with Dose/hr Given

$$\frac{\text{Dose/hr desired}}{\text{Concentration}} = \text{IR in mL/hr}$$

Example: A patient is to receive 1.2 g/hr of aminocaproic acid using a concentration of 15 g aminocaproic acid/500 mL D5W (0.03 g/mL)

$$\frac{\text{1.2 g/hr}}{\text{0.03 g/mL}} = \text{40 mL/hr}$$

To Calculate Infusion Rate (IR) with Dose/min Given

$$\frac{\text{Desired Dose/min} \times \text{60 mL/hr}}{\text{Concentration}} = \text{IR in mL/hr}$$

Example: A patient is to receive 400 µg/min of dopamine using a concentration of 400 mg dopamine/500 mL D5W (800 µg/mL)

$$\frac{\text{400 µg/min x 60 mL/hr}}{\text{800 µg/mL}} = \text{30 mL/hr}$$

To Calculate Infusion Rate (IR) with ug/kg/min Given

$$\frac{\text{Body weight in kg} \times \text{desired dose in µg/kg/min}}{\text{Concentration in µg/mL}} = \textbf{IR (pump setting)}$$

Example: A 60-kg patient is to receive a 10-µg/kg/min dopamine infusion using a concentration of 400 mg/500 mL D5W (800 µg/mL)

$$\frac{60\text{ kg} \times 10\text{ µg/kg/min}}{800\text{ µg/mL}} \times \frac{60\text{ min}}{1\text{ hr}} = \text{IR (pump setting)} = \mathbf{45\ mL/hr}$$

IR = Infusion Rate = Pump Setting = mL/hr

Useful Formulae and Tables

Body Surface Area (BSA) in meters^2 (m^2)

$$BSA = \text{weight (kg)}^{0.425} \times \text{height (cm)}^{0.725} \times 71.84$$

or

$$BSA = (0.061 \times \text{weight [kg]}) \times 0.805$$

Lean Body Weight (LBW) in kg

Males $LBW = \dfrac{1.10 \times \text{weight (kg)} - 128 \times \text{weight}^2 \text{ (kg)}}{\text{height}^2 \text{ (cm)}}$

Females $LBW = \dfrac{1.07 \times \text{weight (kg)} - 148 \times \text{weight}^2 \text{ (kg)}}{\text{height}^2 \text{ (cm)}}$

Creatinine Clearance (Cl_{cr} cc/min)

Males $Cl_{cr} = \dfrac{(140 - \text{age in years}) - \text{body weight (kg)}}{72 \times \text{serum creatinine } (C_{cr})}$

Females $Cl_{cr} = 0.85 \times \dfrac{(140 - \text{age in years}) - \text{body weight (kg)}}{72 \times \text{serum creatinine } (C_{cr})}$

Conversions

1000 nanograms (ng) = 1 microgram (μg)
1000 micrograms (μg) = 1 milligram (mg)
1000 milligrams (mg) = 1 gram (g)
1000 grams (g) = 1 kilogram (kg)

1 kilogram (kg) = 2.2 pounds (lb)
1 pound (lb) = 0.455 kilogram (kg)

1 milliliter (mL) = 1 cubic centimeter (cc)

Temperature (°F) = 9/5 (centigrade temperature) + 32
Temperature (°C) = 5/9 (Fahrenheit temperature − 32)

1 inch (in) = 2.54 centimeters (cm)
1 centimeter (cm) = 0.394 inch (in)

Shargel L, Yu A: *Applied Biopharmaceutics and Pharmacokinetics*, Norwalk, CT Appleton Langer 1993, p. 420.

Fahrenheit to Celsius Conversion Table

Fahrenheit	Celsius	Fahrenheit	Celsius	Fahrenheit	Celsius	Fahrenheit	Celsius	Fahrenheit	Celsius
95.0	35.0	97.0	36.1	99.0	37.2	101.0	38.3	103.0	39.4
95.2	35.1	97.2	36.2	99.2	37.3	101.2	38.4	103.2	39.5
95.4	35.2	97.4	36.3	99.4	37.4	101.4	38.5	103.4	39.6
95.6	35.3	97.6	36.4	99.6	37.5	101.6	38.6	103.6	39.7
95.8	35.4	97.8	36.5	99.8	37.6	101.8	38.7	103.8	39.8
96.0	35.5	98.0	36.6	100.0	37.7	102.0	38.8	104.0	40.0
96.2	35.6	98.2	36.7	100.2	37.8	102.2	39.0	104.2	40.1
96.4	35.7	98.4	36.8	100.4	38.0	102.4	39.1	104.4	40.2
96.6	35.8	98.6	37.0	100.6	38.1	102.6	39.2	104.6	40.3
96.8	36.0	98.8	37.1	100.8	38.2	102.8	39.3	104.8	40.4

Temperature Correction Factors for Blood pH and Gas Measurements (Add to observed value)

Patient's Temperature				
°F	°C	pH	Pco_2 (%)	Po_2 (%)
110	43	−0.09	+22	+35
107	41.5	−0.07	+17	+27
106	41	−0.06	+16	+25
105	40.5	−0.05	+14	+22
104	40	−0.04	+12	+19
103	39.5	−0.04	+10	+16
102	39	−0.03	+ 8	+13
101	38.5	−0.02	+ 6	+10
100	38	−0.01	+ 4	+ 7
98–99	37	None	None	None
97	36	+0.01	− 4	− 7
96	35.5	+0.02	− 6	−10
95	35	+0.03	− 8	−13
94	34.5	+0.04	−10	−16
93	34	+0.04	−12	−19
92	33.5	+0.05	−14	−22
91	33	+0.06	−16	−25
90	32	+0.07	−19	−30
88	31	+0.09	−22	−35
86	30	+0.10	−26	−39
84	29	+0.12	−29	−43
82	28	+0.13	−32	−47
80	26	+0.15	−36	−53
75	24	+0.19	−43	−60

From Marini JJ, Wheeler AP: *Critical Care Medicine—The Essentials.* Baltimore, Williams & Wilkins, 1989, p. 300.

Useful Respiratory Formulae and Normal Values

Quantity	Formula	Normal
Tidal volume (V_T)	6–7 mL/kg	≈ 500 mL
Vital capacity (VC)		65–70 mL/kg
Maximal inspiratory pressure (MIP)		>75–100 cmH_2O
Deadspace (V_O)	≈ 1/2 V_T	1 mL/pound or 0.45 mL/kg
Deadspace ratio (V_O/V_T)	$(Paco_2 - P_Eco_2)/Paco_2$	0.25–0.40
Minute ventilation ($\dot{V}_E$)		5–10 L/min
Maximal ventilatory volume (MVV)	≈ 35 × FEV_1	
Peak flow	(height, age, sex dependent)	> 7L/sec or > 425 L/min
Dynamic characteristic	$V_T/(P_{aw} - PEEP)$	Flow dependent
Static compliance (C_{stat})	$V_T/(P_{plat} - PEEP)$	80 mL/cmH_2O
Resistance to airflow (R_L)	$(P_{dyn} - P_{plat})$/flow	< 4 cmH_2O/L/sec
Alveolar partial pressure of O_2 (P_{AO_2})	$(P_B - PH_2O) \times F_{IO_2} - (Paco_2) / 0.8$	> 100 mmHg
Arterial-alveolar difference ($A\text{-}aDo_2$)	$P_{AO_2} - Pao_2$	<10 mmHg @ $F_{IO_2} = 0.21$
Arterial Pao_2/F_{IO_2} ratio (P/F)	Pao_2/F_{IO_2}	> 400
Arterial/alveolar ratio (a/A)	Pao_2/P_{AO_2}	> 0.9
Arterial O_2 tension (Pao_2)	100 − (age/3)	80–95 mmHg
Arterial O_2 saturation (Sao_2)		Sao_2 > 90%
Arterial CO_2 tension ($PaCo_2$)		37–43 mmHg
Mixed venous O_2 tension ($P\bar{v}O_2$)		≈ 35–40 mmHg

Useful Respiratory Formulae and Normal Values *(continued)*

Quantity	Formula	Normal
Mixed venous O_2 saturation ($S\bar{v}O_2$)		> 70%
Mixed venous CO_2 tension ($P\bar{v}CO_2$)		≈ 45 mmHg
Arterial O_2 content (CaO_2)	$(Hgb \times 1.34)SaO_2 + (PaO_2 \times 0.003)$	≈ 20 mL/dL
Venous O_2 content ($C\bar{v}O_2$)	$(Hgb \times 1.34)\ S\bar{v}O_2 + (P\bar{v}O_2 \times 0.003)$	≈ 15 mL/dL
Oxygen consumption ($\dot{V}O_2$)	$CO_1 \times C(a\text{-}v)O_{2\,mL/dL} \times 10$	≈ 250 mL/min
Extraction ratio	$C(a\text{-}\dot{v})O_2/CaO_2)$	≈ 0.25
Pulmonary capillary O_2 content (CcO_2)	$(Hgb \times 1.34) + (PAO_2 \times 0.003)$	≈ 20 mL/dL
Shunt fraction (venous admixture) % ($\dot{Q}_s / \dot{Q}_T$)	$(CcO_2 - CaO_2)/(CcO_2 - C\bar{v}O_2) \times 100$	< 5%
Arteriovenous O_2 content difference $C(a\text{-}\bar{v})O_2$	$CaO_2 - C\bar{v}O_2$	≈ 5 mL/dL

From Marini JJ, Wheeler AP: *Critical Care Medicine—The Essentials.* Baltimore, Williams & Wilkins, 1989, p. 299.

Useful Renal Formulae and Normal Values*

Quantity	Formula	Normal
Estimated creatinine clearance (Cl_{Cr})	$\frac{(140 - \text{age})(\text{wt in kg})}{72 \times \text{serum [Cr]}}$	>100 mL/min
Renal failure index (RFI)	$\frac{\text{Urine }[Na^+] \times \text{serum [Cr]}}{\text{Urine [Cr]}}$	<1 Prerenal >1 Intrarenal
Fractional excretion of sodium (FENa)	$\frac{(\text{Urine }[Na^+] \times \text{serum [Cr]})}{(\text{Serum }[Na^+] \times \text{urine [Cr]})} \times 100$	<1 Prerenal >1 Intrarenal
Anion gap (AG)	$[Na^+] - ([Cl^-] + [HCO_3^-])$	8–12 mEq/L
Calculated osmolality (Osm)	$2 \times [Na^+]$ + [glucose]/18 + [BUN]/2.8	285–295 mOsm/L
Calculated H_2O deficit (liters)	0.6 (wt in kg) $\times$ ($[Na^+]$ − 140)/140	
Corrected $[Ca^{2+}]$	If albumin ↓ by 1 g/dL $[Ca^{2+}]$ ↓ by 0.8 mg/dL	
Colloid osmotic pressure (COP)	1.4 [globulin]* + 5.5 [albumin]*	24 ± 3 mmHg

*wt, weight; ↑, increased; ↓, decreased; *, (g/dL).
From Marini JJ, Wheeler AP: *Critical Care Medicine—The Essentials.* Baltimore, Williams & Wilkins, 1989, p. 277.

Content of Common Intravenous Fluids

Type	Electrolytes (mEq/L)						Calories and Osmolality	
	Na^+	Cl^-	K^+	Ca^{2+}	Lactate	HCO_3^-	mOsm/L	kcal/L
D5W	0	0	0	0	0	0	252	170
D50W	0	0	0	0	0	0	2530	1700
1/2 NS	77	77	0	0	0	0	154	0
NS	154	154	0	0	0	0	308	0
Ringer's lactate	130	109	4	3	28	0	273	0
3% NaCl	513	513	0	0	0	0	1026	0
D5 1/2NS	77	77	0	0	0	0	406	170
$NaHCO_3$	1000					1000	2000	0
20% Mannitol	0	0	0	0	0	0	1098	

From Marini JJ, Wheeler AP: *Critical Care Medicine—The Essentials.* Baltimore, Williams & Wilkins, 1989, p. 299.

Composition and Properties of Colloidal Solutions*

Solution	Volume(s) (mL)	Composition (mEq/L)			pH	Tonicity Relative to Plasma	Osmolarity (mOsm/L)
		Sodium	Chloride	Calcium			
5% Albumin	250, 500	145	145	0	6.9	Isotonic	~300
25% Albumin	20, 50, 100	145	145	0	6.9	Hypertonic	?
Plasma protein fraction	250, 500	145	145	0	7.0	Isotonic	~300
6% Hetastarch	500	154	154	0	5.5	Isotonic	310
10% Pentastarch	500	154	154	0	5.0	Isotonic	326
10% Dextran 40	500	0/154†	0/154†	0	4.5	Isotonic	300
6% Dextran 70	500	0/154	0/154	0	4.5	Isotonic	300
6% Dextran 75	500	0/154	0/154	0	4.5	Isotonic	300
Modified fluid gelatin	500	154	125	0	7.4	Isotonic	279
Polygeline	500	145	145	12	7.3	Isotonic	370
Oxypolygelatin	250,500	154	130	1	7.0	Isotonic	300

*All colloidal solutions are preservative free.

†Dextrans are available both in 0.9% sodium chloride injection and in 5% dextrose injection.

Originally published in Composition and properties of colloidal solutions.

Blood Products

Blood Product	Volume (mL)	Contents	Comments
Whole Blood	510	450 mL blood 60 mL CPD	No viable platelets after 24 hours. K^+ accumulates after a few days
Packed RBCs	300	200 mL cells 100 mL plasma	Hct usually 60 to 70, and must be diluted with saline
Plasma	240	All clotting factors	Used for clotting factors. Not used as plasma expander
Platelet concentrate	50	50×10^{10} platelets	Outdated after 72 hours
Cryoprecipitate	20	200 mg fibrinogen 100 µg Factor VIII 150 µg VWF	Rich in fibronectin Expensive and has little use in the ICU

CPD, citrate phosphate dextrose; VWF, von Willebrand factor.
From Marino PL: *The ICU Book.* Malvern, PA, Lea & Febiger, 1991, p. 656.

Normal Resting Hemodynamic Pressures

	Systolic	End-Diastolic	Mean
Right atrium (RA)			2–8
Right ventricle (RV)	15–30	2–8	
Pulmonary artery (PA)	15–30	4–12	9–18
Pulmonary capillary wedge (PCW)			2–10
Left atrium (LA)			2–10
Left ventricle (LV)	100–140	3–12	
Systemic artery	100–140	60–90	70–105

From Grossman W (ed): *Cardiac Catheterization and Angiography.* Philadelphia, Lea & Febiger, 1986.

Hemodynamic Formulae

Parameter	Formula	Units	Normal Value
Arterial oxygen content	$C_A = 0.0031 \times$ arterial $Po_2 + 1.38 \times$ Hb $\times$ arterial oxygen saturation (Sao_2)	Vol %	20.4
Arterial oxygen saturation		%	97–100
Cardiac index	$CI = \frac{CO}{BSA}$	$L/min/M^2$	2.6–4.2
Cardiac output (Fick)	$CO = \frac{Vo_2}{Cao_2 - C\bar{v}o_2}$	L/min	5.4 ± 1.2
Central blood volume	CBV = Mean transit time $\times$ CI $\times$ 16.7	$mL/m^{\%}$	830 ± 86
Central venous pressure	$CVP = \frac{\text{Water CVP (cm)}}{1.36}$	mmHg	2–8
Circulating blood volume	$\simeq$70 ml/kg	mL	$\simeq$5000 ml
Ejection fraction (EF)	SV/end-diastolic volume	%	LV 65$\pm$5; RV 55$\pm$5
Heart rate max (HR_{max})	220 $-$ age		
Left ventricular stroke work	LVSW = CI $\times$ MAP $\times$ 0.144	$kg/m/m^2$	3.8 ± 0.4
Left ventricular stroke work index	LVSWI = SI $\times$ MAP $\times$ 0.144	$g/m/m^2$	56 ± 6
Mean arterial pressure	$MAP = \frac{2(\text{diastolic}) + \text{systolic}}{3}$	mmHg	70–105
Oxygen consumption	$VO_2 = CI \times Hb \times 13.8 \times (Sao_2 - S\bar{v}o_2)$	$L/min/M^2$	110–150
Oxygen delivery (Do_2)	CI $\times$ CaO_2	$\simeq$700 mL $O_2/min/m^2$	520–720
Oxygen extraction ratio	$o_2ER = 1 - \frac{Vo_2}{Do_2} \times 100$	%	22–32

Oxygen uptake	$Vo_2 = CI \times (Cao_2 - Cvo_2)$	mL/min/m^2	110–160
Pulmonary artery saturation		%	75%
Pulmonary vascular resistance	$PVR = \left(\frac{\text{mean PA pressure} - \text{mean LA or PCW pressure}}{CO}\right) \times 80$	dynes-sec-cm^{-5}	67 ± 30
Pulmonary vascular resistance index	$PVRI = \frac{PVR}{BSA}$	dynes-sec-cm^{-5} • M^2	123 ± 54
Right ventricular stroke work	$RVSW = CI \times MPAP \times 0.144$	kg/m/m^2	0.6 ± 0.06
Right ventricular stroke work index	$RVSWI = SI \times MPAP \times 0.144$	g/m/m^2	8.8 ± 0.9
Stroke index	$SI = \frac{CI}{HR} \times 1000$	mL/beat/M^2	30–65
Stroke volume	$SV = \frac{CO}{HR}$	mL/beat	70–130
Systemic vascular resistance	$SVR = \left(\frac{MAP - \text{mean RA pressure}}{CO}\right) \times 80$	dynes-sec-cm^{-5}	1170 ± 270
Systemic vascular resistance index	$SVRI = \frac{SVR}{BSA}$	dynes-sec-cm^{-5} • M^2	2180 ± 210
Total pulmonary resistance	$TPR = \left(\frac{\text{mean PA pressure}}{CO}\right) \times 80$	dynes-sec-cm^{-5}	200 ± 50
Venous oxygen content	$C\bar{v}O_2 = 0.0031 \times \text{venous } Po_2 + 1.38 \times Hb \times \text{venous oxygen saturation } (S\bar{v}o_2)$	Vol %	15.1

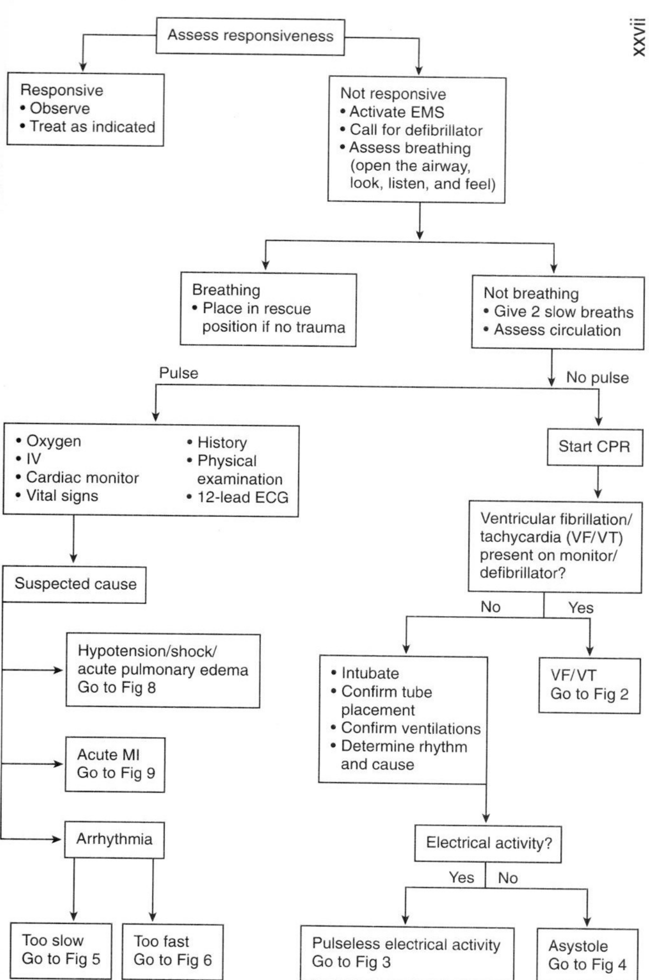

Fig. 1. Universal algorithm for adult emergency cardiac care. (From Emergency Cardiac Care Committee and Subcommittees, American Heart Association, American Heart Association. Guidelines for Cardiopulmonary Resuscitation and Emergency Cardiac Care. JAMA 268(16): 2171-2195, 1992. Copyright 1992, American Medical Association.)

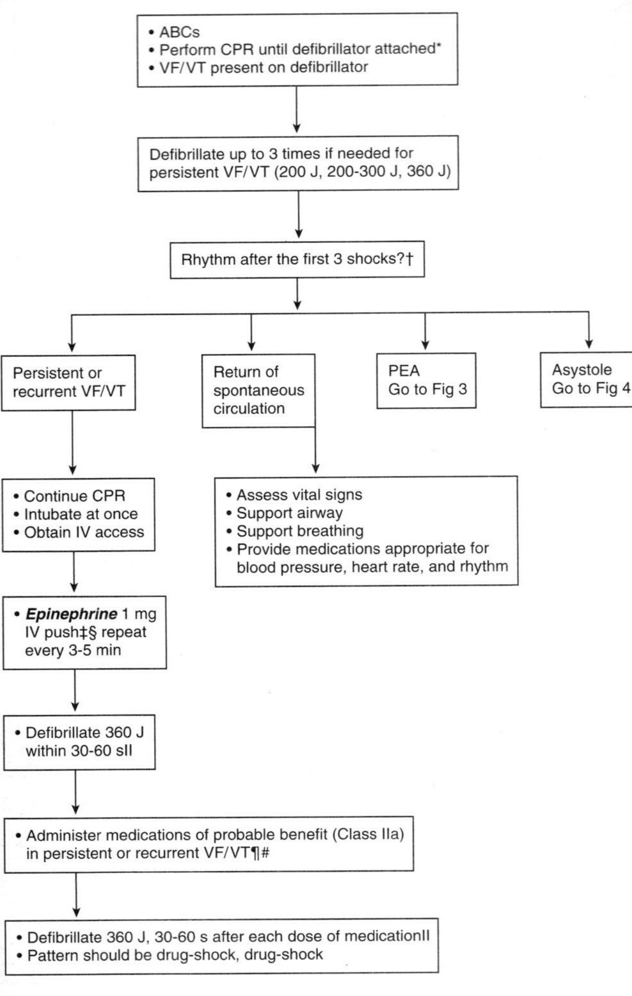
• ABCs
• Perform CPR until defibrillator attached*
• VF/VT present on defibrillator
Defibrillate up to 3 times if needed for persistent VF/VT (200 J, 200-300 J, 360 J)
Rhythm after the first 3 shocks?†
Persistent or recurrent VF/VT
Return of spontaneous circulation
PEA Go to Fig 3
Asystole Go to Fig 4
• Continue CPR
• Intubate at once
• Obtain IV access
• Assess vital signs
• Support airway
• Support breathing
• Provide medications appropriate for blood pressure, heart rate, and rhythm
• Epinephrine 1 mg IV push‡§ repeat every 3-5 min
• Defibrillate 360 J within 30-60 sII
• Administer medications of probable benefit (Class IIa) in persistent or recurrent VF/VT¶#
• Defibrillate 360 J, 30-60 s after each dose of medicationII
• Pattern should be drug-shock, drug-shock

Class I: definitely helpful
Class IIa: acceptable, probably helpful
Class IIb: acceptable, possibly helpful
Class III: not indicated, may be harmful

* Precordial thump is a Class IIb action in witnessed arrest, no pulse, and no defibrillator immediately available.

† Hypothermic cardiac arrest is treated differently after this point. See section on hypothermia.

‡ The recommended dose of ***epinephrine*** is 1 mg IV push every 3-5 min. If this approach fails, several Class IIb dosing regimens can be considered:
- Intermediate: ***epinephrine*** 2-5 mg IV push, every 3-5 min
- Escalating: ***epinephrine*** 1 mg-3 mg-5 mg IV push (3 min apart)
- High: ***epinephrine*** 0.1 mg/kg IV push, every 3-5 min

§ ***Sodium bicarbonate*** (1 mEq/kg) is Class I if patient has known preexisting hyperkalemia

II Multiple sequenced shocks (200 J, 200-300 J, 360 J) are acceptable here (Class I), especially when medications are delayed

¶
- ***Lidocaine*** 1.5 mg/kg IV push. Repeat in 3-5 min to total loading dose of 3 mg/kg; then use
- ***Bretylium*** 5 mg/kg IV push. Repeat in 5 min at 10 mg/kg
- ***Magnesium sulfate*** 1-2 g IV in torsades de pointes or suspected hypomagnesemic state or severe refractory VF
- ***Procainamide*** 30 mg/min in refractory VF (maximum total 17 mg/kg)

\#
- ***Sodium bicarbonate*** (1 mEq/kg IV):

Class IIa
- if known preexisting bicarbonate-responsive acidosis
- if overdose with tricyclic antidepressants
- to alkalinize the urine in drug overdoses

Class IIb
- if intubated and continued long arrest interval
- upon return of spontaneous circulation after long arrest interval

Class III
- hypoxic lactic acidosis

Fig. 2. Algorithm for ventricular fibrillation and pulseless ventricular tachycardia (VFNT). (From Emergency Cardiac Care Committee and Subcommittees, American Heart Association, American Heart Association. Guidelines for Cardiopulmonary Resuscitation and Emergency Cardiac Care. JAMA 268(16): 2171-2195, 1992. Copyright 1992, American Medical Association.)

PEA includes
- Electromechanical dissociation (EMD)
- Pseudo-EMD
- Idioventricular rhythms
- Ventricular escape rhythms
- Bradyasystolic rhythms
- Postdefibrillation idioventricular rhythms

↓

- Continue CPR
- Intubate at once
- Obtain IV access
- Assess blood flow using Doppler ultrasound

↓

Consider possible causes
(Parentheses = possible therapies and treatments)
- Hypovolemia (volume infusion)
- Hypoxia (ventilation)
- Cardiac tamponade (pericardiocentesis)
- Tension pneumothorax (needle decompression)
- Hypothermia (see hypothermia algorithm, Fig 11)
- Massive pulmonary embolism (surgery, ***thrombolytics***)
- Drug overdoses such as tricyclics, digitalis, β-blockers, calcium channel blockers
- Hyperkalemia*
- Acidosis†
- Massive acute myocardial infarction (go to Fig 9)

↓

- ***Epinephrine*** 1 mg IV push,*‡ repeat every 3-5 min

↓

- If absolute bradycardia (<60 beats/min) or relative bradycardia, give ***atropine*** 1 mg IV
- Repeat every 3-5 min up to a total of 0.04 mg/kg§

Class I: definitely helpful
Class IIa: acceptable, probably helpful
Class IIb: acceptable, possibly helpful
Class III: not indicated, may be harmful

* ***Sodium bicarbonate*** 1 mEq/kg is Class I if patient has known preexisting hyperkalemia

† ***Sodium bicarbonate*** 1 mEq/kg:
Class IIa
- if known preexisting bicarbonate-responsive acidosis
- if overdose with tricyclic antidepressants
- to alkalinize the urine in drug overdoses

Class IIb
- if intubated and long arrest interval
- upon return of spontaneous circulation after long arrest interval

Class III
- hypoxic lactic acidosis

‡ The recommended dose of ***epinephrine*** is 1 mg IV push every 3-5 min.
If this approach fails, several Class IIb dosing regimens can be considered.
- Intermediate: ***epinephrine*** 2-5 mg IV push, every 3-5 min
- Escalating: ***epinephrine*** 1 mg-3 mg-5 mg IV push (3 min apart)
- High: ***epinephrine*** 0.1 mg/kg IV push, every 3-5 min

§ Shorter ***atropine*** dosing intervals are possibly helpful in cardiac arrest (Class IIb).

Fig. 3. Algorithm for pulseless electrical activity (PEA) (electromechanical dissociation [EMD]). (From Emergency Cardiac Care Committee and Subcommittees, American Heart Association, American Heart Association. Guidelines for Cardiopulmonary Resuscitation and Emergency Cardiac Care. JAMA 268(16): 2171-2195, 1992. Copyright 1992, American Medical Association.)

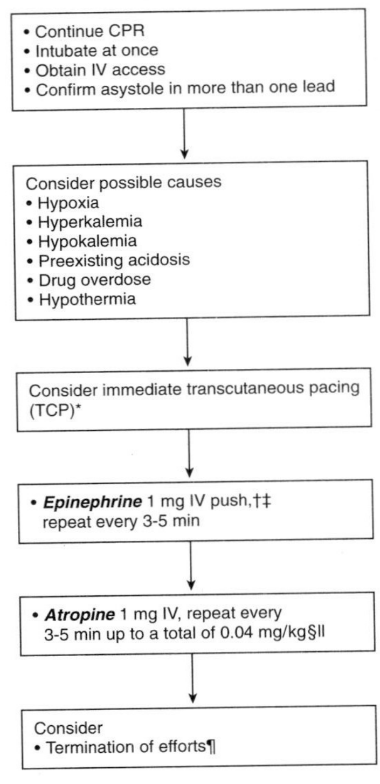
• Continue CPR
• Intubate at once
• Obtain IV access
• Confirm asystole in more than one lead
Consider possible causes
• Hypoxia
• Hyperkalemia
• Hypokalemia
• Preexisting acidosis
• Drug overdose
• Hypothermia
Consider immediate transcutaneous pacing (TCP)*
• Epinephrine 1 mg IV push,†‡ repeat every 3-5 min
• Atropine 1 mg IV, repeat every 3-5 min up to a total of 0.04 mg/kg§ll
Consider
• Termination of efforts¶

Class I: definitely helpful
Class IIa: acceptable, probably helpful
Class IIb: acceptable, possibly helpful
Class III: not indicated, may be harmful

* TCP is a Class IIb intervention. Lack of success may be due to delay in pacing. To be effective TCP must be performed early, simultaneously with drugs. Evidence does not support routine use of TCP for asystole.

† The recommended dose of ***epinephrine*** is 1 mg IV push every 3-5 min. If this approach fails, several Class IIb dosing regimens can be considered:
- Intermediate: ***epinephrine*** 2-5 mg IV push, every 3-5 min
- Escalating: ***epinephrine*** 1 mg-3 mg-5 mg IV push (3 min apart)
- High: ***epinephrine*** 0.1 mg/kg IV push, every 3-5 min

‡ ***Sodium bicarbonate*** 1 mEq/kg is Class I if patient has known preexisting hyperkalemia.

§ Shorter ***atropine*** dosing intervals are Class IIb in asystolic arrest.

II • ***Sodium bicarbonate*** 1 mEq/kg:
Class IIa
- if known preexisting bicarbonate-responsive acidosis
- if overdose with tricyclic antidepressants
- to alkalinize the urine in drug overdose

Class IIb
- if intubated and continued long arrest interval
- upon return of spontaneous circulation after long arrest interval

Class III
- hypoxic lactic acidosis

¶ If patient remains in asystole or other agonal rhythms after successful intubation and initial medication and no reversible causes are identified, consider termination of resuscitative efforts by a physician. Consider interval since arrest.

Fig. 4. Asystole treatment algorithm. (From Emergency Cardiac Care Committee and Subcommittees, American Heart Association, American Heart Association. Guidelines for Cardiopulmonary Resuscitation and Emergency Cardiac Care. JAMA 268(16): 2171-2195, 1992. Copyright 1992, American Medical Association.)

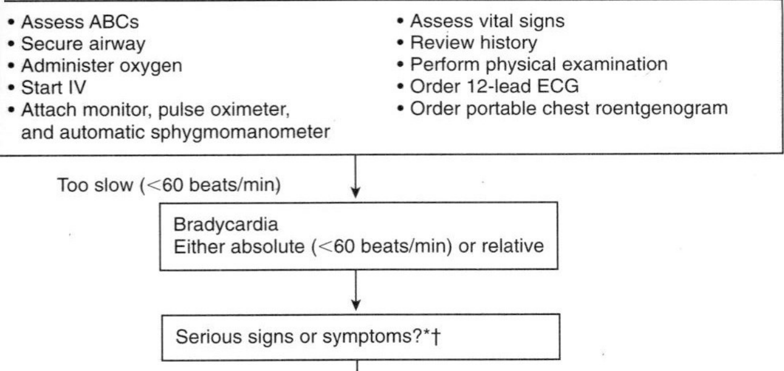

• Assess ABCs
• Secure airway
• Administer oxygen
• Start IV
• Attach monitor, pulse oximeter, and automatic sphygmomanometer
• Assess vital signs
• Review history
• Perform physical examination
• Order 12-lead ECG
• Order portable chest roentgenogram
Too slow (<60 beats/min)
Bradycardia
Either absolute (<60 beats/min) or relative

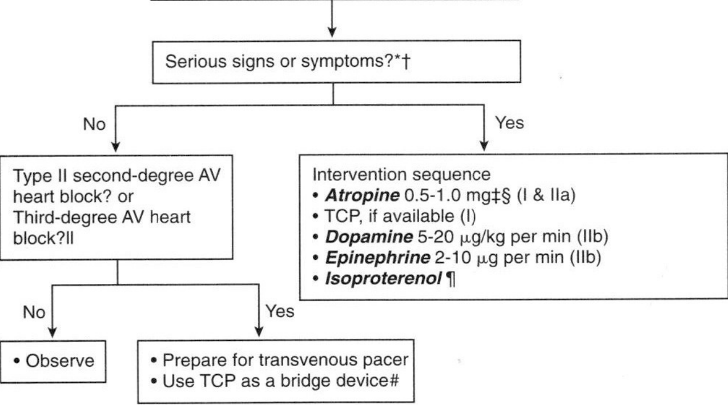

* Serious signs or symptoms must be related to the slow rate. Clinical manifestations include: *symptoms* (chest pain, shortness of breath, decreased level of consciousness) and *signs* (low BP, shock, pulmonary congestion, CHF, acute MI).

† Do not delay TCP while awaiting IV access or for ***atropine*** to take effect if patient is symptomatic.

‡ Denervated transplanted hearts will not respond to ***atropine.*** Go at once to pacing, ***catecholamine*** infusion, or both.

§ ***Atropine*** should be given in repeat doses in 3-5 min up to a total of 0.04 mg/kg. Consider shorter dosing intervals in severe clinical conditions. It has been suggested that atropine should be used with caution in atrioventricular (AV) block at the His-Purkinje level (type II AV block and new third-degree block with wide QRS complexes) (Class IIb).

ll Never treat third-degree heart block plus ventricular escape beats with ***lidocaine.***

¶ ***Isoproterenol*** should be used, if at all, with extreme caution. At low doses it is Class IIb (possibly helpful); at higher doses it is Class III (harmful).

\# Verify patient tolerance and mechanical capture. Use analgesia and sedation as needed.

Fig. 5. Bradycardia algorithm (with the patient not in cardiac arrest). (From Emergency Cardiac Care Committee and Subcommittees, American Heart Association, American Heart Association. Guidelines for Cardiopulmonary Resuscitation and Emergency Cardiac Care. JAMA 268(16): 2171-2195, 1992. Copyright 1992, American Medical Association.)

Indications for Emergent and Standby Pacing

Emergent Pacing
Hemodynamically compromising bradycardias* (Blood pressure <80 mm Hg systolic, change in mental status, myocardial ischemia, pulmonary edema) Bradycardia with malignant escape rhythms (Unresponsive to pharmacological therapy) Overdrive pacing of refractory tachycardia Supraventricular or ventricular (currently indicated only in special situations refractory to pharmacological therapy or cardioversion)
Bradyasystolic Cardiac Arrest
Pacing not routinely recommended in such patients. If used at all, pacing should be used as early as possible after onset of arrest

Stable bradycardias
(Blood pressure >80 mm Hg, no evidence of hemodynamic compromise, or hemodynamic compromise responsive to initial drug therapy)
Prophylactic pacing in acute myocardial infarction
Symptomatic sinus node dysfunction
Mobitz II second-degree heart block
Third-degree heart block
Newly acquired: left bundle-branch block, right bundle-branch block, alternating bundle-branch block, or bifascicular block

*Include complete heart block, symptomatic second-degree heart block, symptomatic sick sinus syndrome, drug-induced bradycardias (i.e., digoxin, beta-blockers, calcium channel blockers, or procainamide), permanent pacemaker failure, idioventricular bradycardias, symptomatic atrial fibrillation with slow ventricular response, refractory bradycardia during resuscitation of hypovolemic shock, and bradyarrhythmias with malignant ventricular escape mechanisms.

From Emergency Cardiac Care Committee and Subcommittees, American Heart Association, American Heart Association. Guidelines for Cardiopulmonary Resuscitation and Emergency Cardiac Care. JAMA 268(16): 2171–2195, 1992. Copyright 1992, American Medical Association.

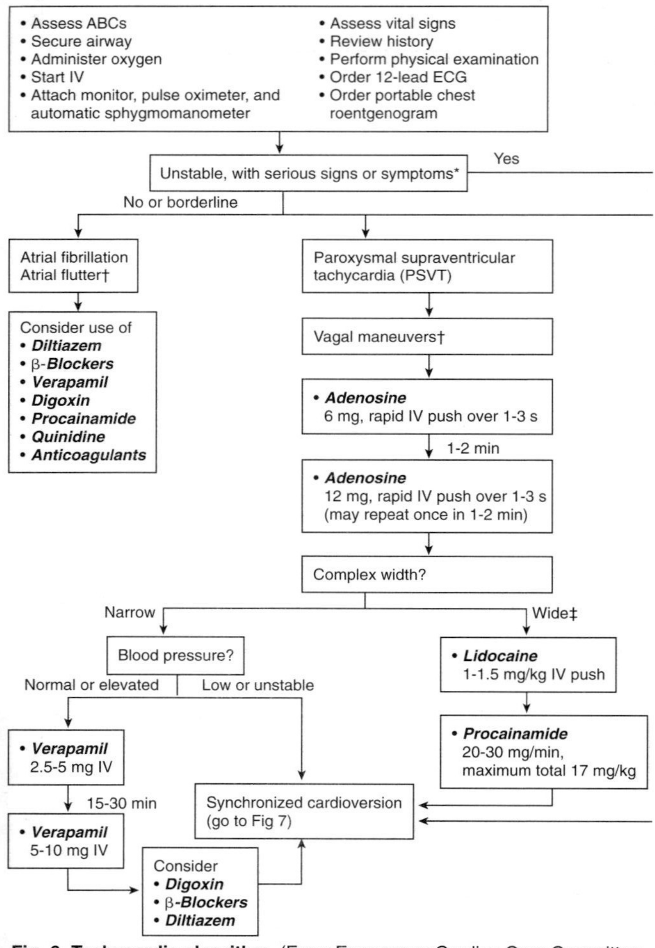

Fig. 6. Tachycardia algorithm. (From Emergency Cardiac Care Committee and Subcommittees, American Heart Association, American Heart Association. Guidelines for Cardiopulmonary Resuscitation and Emergency Cardiac Care. JAMA 268(16): 2171–2195, 1992. Copyright 1992, American Medical Association.)

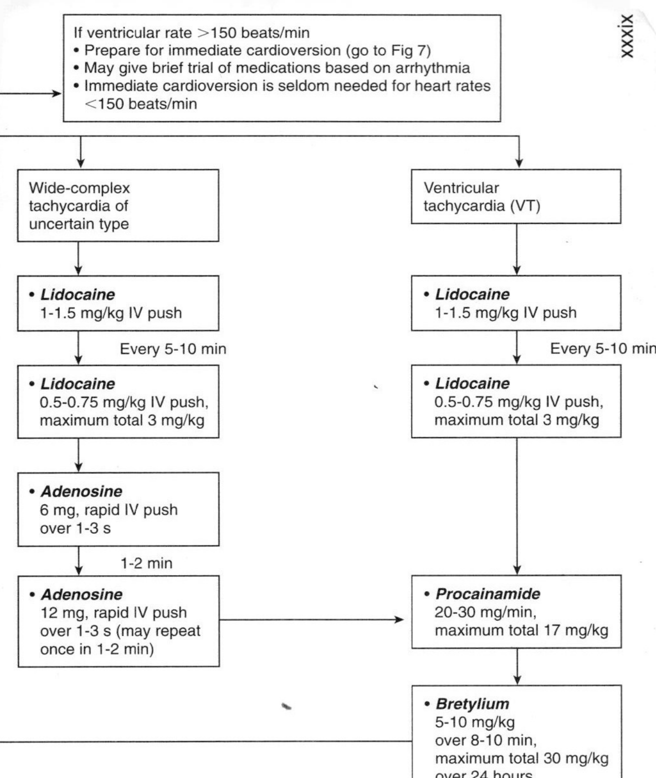

* Unstable condition must be related to the tachycardia. Signs and symptoms may include chest pain, shortness of breath, decreased level of consciousness, low blood pressure (BP), shock, pulmonary congestion, congestive heart failure, acute myocardial infarction.

† Carotid sinus pressure is contraindicated in patients with carotid bruits; avoid ice water immersion in patients with ischemic heart disease.

‡ If the wide-complex tachycardia is known with certainty to be PSVT and BP is normal/elevated, sequence can include ***verapamil.***

Fig. 6. (continued)

Tachycardia with serious signs and symptoms related to the tachycardia

If ventricular rate is >150 beats/min, prepare for immediate cardioversion. May give brief trial of medications based on specific arrhythmias. Immediate cardioversion is generally not needed for rates <150 beats/min.

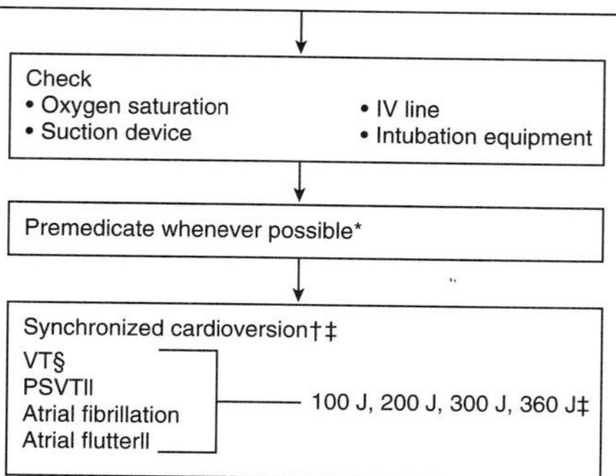

Check
• Oxygen saturation
• Suction device
• IV line
• Intubation equipment
Premedicate whenever possible*
Synchronized cardioversion†‡
VT§
PSVT‖
Atrial fibrillation
Atrial flutter‖
100 J, 200 J, 300 J, 360 J‡

* Effective regimens have included a sedative (eg, ***diazepam, midazolam, barbiturates, etomidate, ketamine, methohexital***) with or without an analgesic agent (eg, ***fentanyl, morphine, meperidine***). Many experts recommend anesthesia if service is readily available.
† Note possible need to resynchronize after each cardioversion.
‡ If delays in synchronization occur and clinical conditions are critical, go to immediate unsynchronized shocks.
§ Treat polymorphic VT (irregular form and rate) like VF: 200 J, 200-300 J, 360 J.
‖ PSVT and atrial flutter often respond to lower energy levels (start with 50 J).

Fig. 7. Electrical cardioversion algorithm (with the patient not in cardiac arrest). (From Emergency Cardiac Care Committee and Subcommittees, American Heart Association, American Heart Association. Guidelines for Cardiopulmonary Resuscitation and Emergency Cardiac Care. JAMA 268(16): 2171–2195, 1992. Copyright 1992, American Medical Association.)

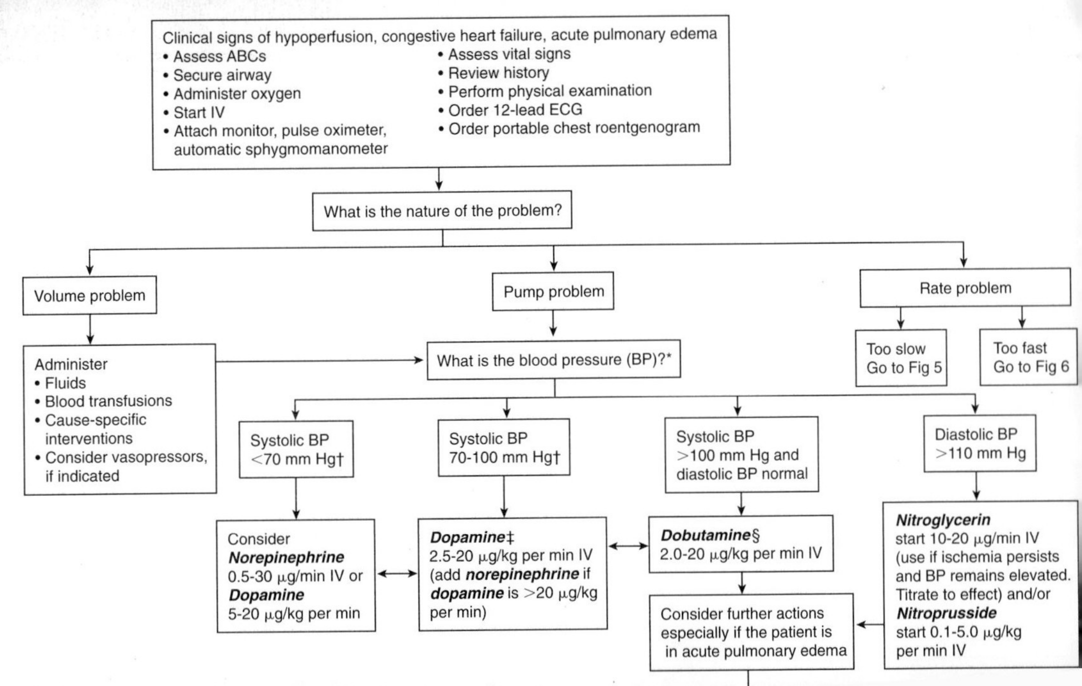

Clinical signs of hypoperfusion, congestive heart failure, acute pulmonary edema
• Assess ABCs
• Secure airway
• Administer oxygen
• Start IV
• Attach monitor, pulse oximeter, automatic sphygmomanometer
• Assess vital signs
• Review history
• Perform physical examination
• Order 12-lead ECG
• Order portable chest roentgenogram
What is the nature of the problem?
Volume problem
Pump problem
Rate problem
Too slow Go to Fig 5
Too fast Go to Fig 6
Administer
• Fluids
• Blood transfusions
• Cause-specific interventions
• Consider vasopressors, if indicated
What is the blood pressure (BP)?*
Systolic BP <70 mm Hg†
Systolic BP 70-100 mm Hg†
Systolic BP >100 mm Hg and diastolic BP normal
Diastolic BP >110 mm Hg
Consider Norepinephrine 0.5-30 μg/min IV or Dopamine 5-20 μg/kg per min
Dopamine‡ 2.5-20 μg/kg per min IV (add norepinephrine if dopamine is >20 μg/kg per min)
Dobutamine§ 2.0-20 μg/kg per min IV
Nitroglycerin start 10-20 μg/min IV (use if ischemia persists and BP remains elevated. Titrate to effect) and/or Nitroprusside start 0.1-5.0 μg/kg per min IV
Consider further actions especially if the patient is in acute pulmonary edema

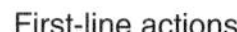

First-line actions
- ***Furosemide*** IV 0.5-1.0 mg/kg
- ***Morphine*** IV 1-3 mg
- ***Nitroglycerin*** SL
- Oxygen/intubate PRN

Second-line actions
- ***Nitroglycerin*** IV (if BP >100 mm Hg)
- ***Nitroprusside*** IV (if BP >100 mm Hg)
- ***Dopamine*** (if BP <100 mm Hg)
- ***Dobutamine*** (if BP >100 mm Hg)
- Positive end-expiratory pressure (PEEP)
- Continuous positive airway pressure (CPAP)

Third-line actions
- ***Amrinone*** 0.75 mg/kg then 5-15 μg/kg per min (if other drugs fail)
- ***Aminophylline*** 5 mg/kg (if wheezing)
- ***Thrombolytic*** therapy (if not in shock)
- ***Digoxin*** (if atrial fibrillation, supraventricular tachycardias)
- Angioplasty (if drugs fail)
- Intra-aortic balloon pump (bridge to surgery)
- Surgical interventions (valves, coronary artery bypass grafts, heart transplant)

* Base management after this point on invasive hemodynamic monitoring if possible.
† Fluid bolus of 250-500 mL normal saline should be tried. If no response, consider sympathomimetics.
‡ Move to ***dopamine*** and stop ***norepinephrine*** when BP improves.
§ Add ***dopamine*** when BP improves. Avoid ***dobutamine*** when systolic BP <100 mm Hg.

Fig. 8. Algorithm for hypotension, shock, and acute pulmonary edema. (From Emergency Cardiac Care Committee and Subcommittees, American Heart Association, American Heart Association. Guidelines for Cardiopulmonary Resuscitation and Emergency Cardiac Care. JAMA 268(16): 2171–2195, 1992. Copyright 1992, American Medical Association.)

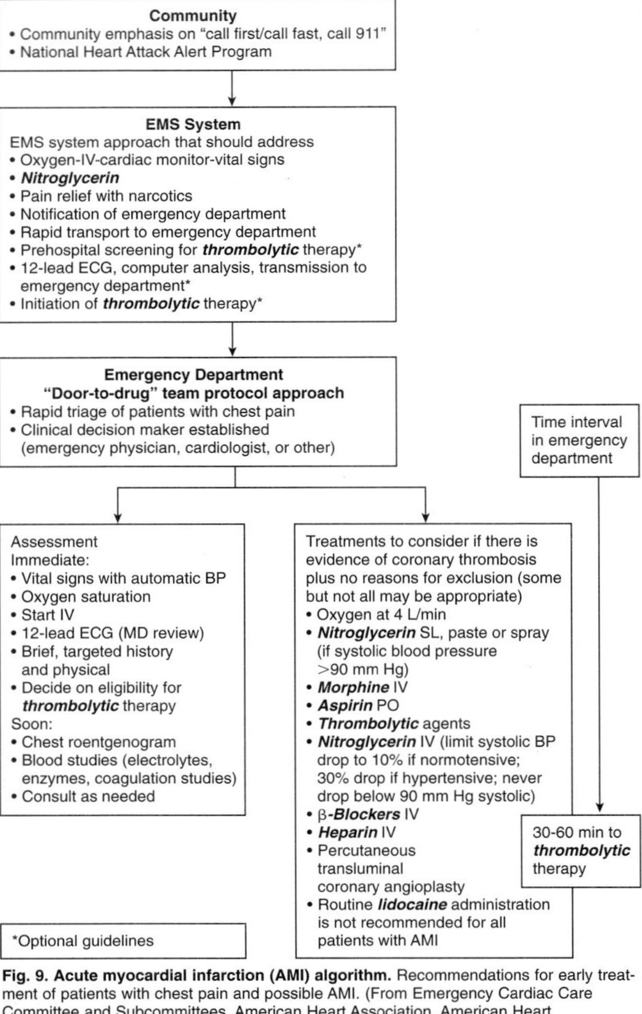

Fig. 9. Acute myocardial infarction (AMI) algorithm. Recommendations for early treatment of patients with chest pain and possible AMI. (From Emergency Cardiac Care Committee and Subcommittees, American Heart Association, American Heart Association. Guidelines for Cardiopulmonary Resuscitation and Emergency Cardiac Care. JAMA 268(16): 2171–2195, 1992. Copyright 1992, American Medical Association.)

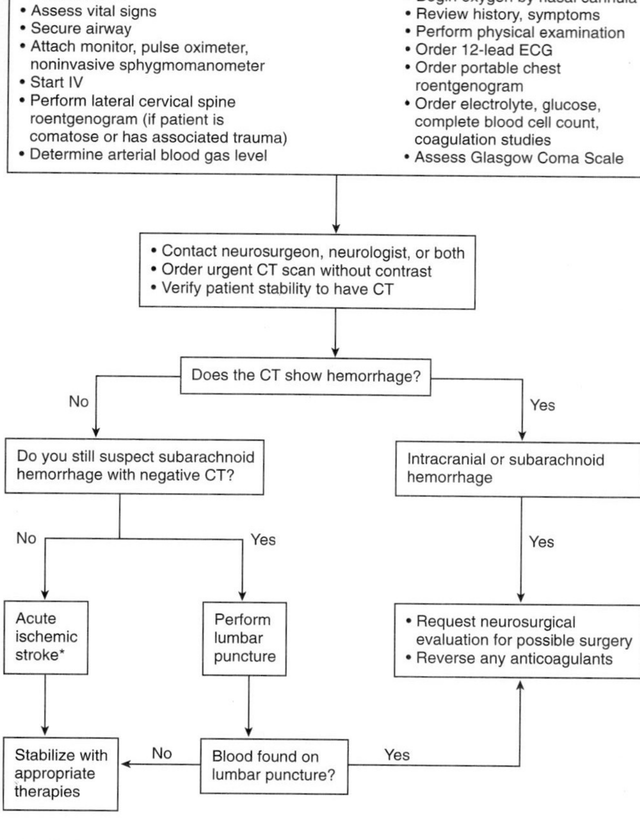

*The detailed management of acute stroke is beyond the scope of the ACLS program. Management of cardiovascular emergencies in stroke victims is similar to the management in other patients. Never forget, however, that acute stroke can coexist with acute cardiovascular problems.

Fig. 10. Algorithm for initial evaluation of suspected stroke. (From Emergency Cardiac Care Committee and Subcommittees, American Heart Association, American Heart Association. Guidelines for Cardiopulmonary Resuscitation and Emergency Cardiac Care. JAMA 268(16): 2171–2195, 1992. Copyright 1992, American Medical Association.)

Emergency Treatment of a Stroke Patient*

Contact neurologist or neurosurgeon
Fluid management (Class IIa[†])
  Intravenous access
  Normal saline or lactated Ringer's at 30 mL/h
  Measure intake and output
  Slow infusion rate
Antihypertensive drugs: computed tomography–guided therapy (class IIa)
  Use rarely and cautiously in ischemic stroke
  Lower blood pressure to estimated prestroke levels in hemorrhagic stroke
Anticonvulsants (class I)
  Phenytoin (15 mg/kg for adults) orally or IV; give no faster than 50 mg/min if administered IV
  Diazepam (10 mg IV for adults)
  Phenobarbital (15 mg/kg IV); use caution for respiratory depression
Treatment of increased intracranial pressure (class I)
  Fluid restriction
  Intubation and hyperventilation to a P_{CO_2} of 25–28 mmHg
  Mannitol support (1–2 g/kg IV over 5–10 minutes)
  Drainage of cerebrospinal fluid by intraventricular catheter
  Surgical intervention

Other interventions
- Surgery (class I)
  - Clip aneurysm
  - Resect arteriovenous malformation
  - Evaluate hematoma
- Nimodipine for subarachnoid hemorrhage (class I)
- Anticoagulants (class IIb‡)
- Thrombolytic drugs (class IIb‡)
- New treatments for ischemic stroke‡

---

*Class I, always acceptable, definitely effective; class IIa, probably helpful; class IIb, possibly helpful; Class III, possibly harmful, not indicated.
†Class III if evidence of cerebral edema.
‡Class III if evidence of hemorrhage.
From Emergency Cardiac Care Committee and Subcommittees, American Heart Association, American Heart Association. Guidelines for Cardiopulmonary Resuscitation and Emergency Cardiac Care. JAMA 268(16): 2171–2195, 1992. Copyright 1992, American Medical Association.

Initial Evaluation of a Patient with Acute Stroke

Computed tomography scan of the brain without contrast material
ECG
Chest roentgenogram
Lateral cervical spine roentgenogram
  (patients who are comatose or who have cervical spine pain or tenderness)
Hematologic studies
  Complete blood cell count
  Platelet count
  Prothrombin time
  Partial thromboplastin time
Serum electrolyte determinations (Na, K, Cl, bicarbonate)
Blood glucose level
Other chemical analyses
Arterial blood gas levels

From Emergency Cardiac Care Committee and Subcommittees, American Heart Association, American Heart Association. Guidelines for Cardiopulmonary Resuscitation and Emergency Cardiac Care. JAMA 268(16): 2171–2195, 1992.

Drugs That Can Be Administered Endotracheally

Drug	Dose (mg)	Volume (mL)
Naloxone	0.4–4	10
Atropine	0.5–1	10
Valium	5–10	10
Epinephrine (1:1000)	2–2.5	10
Lidocaine	100	10

Employ 2–2.5 times initial IV dose and dilute in 10 mL distilled water or normal saline.

Instill via catheter beyond tip of endotracheal tube.

Withhold chest compressions and do not nebulize. Follow with several quick insufflations.

From Marino PL: *The ICU Book.* Malvern, PA, Lea & Febiger, 1991, p. 656.

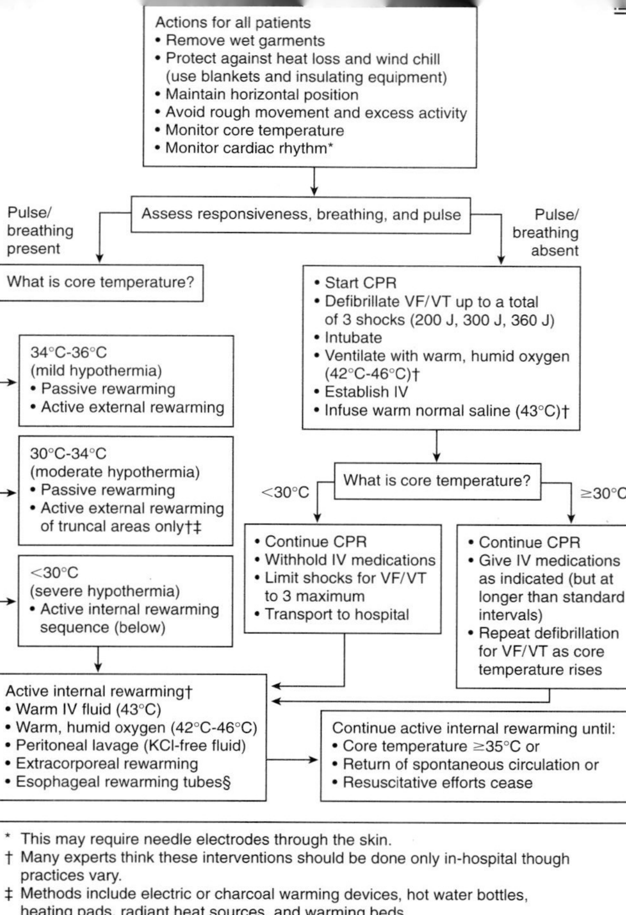
Actions for all patients
• Remove wet garments
• Protect against heat loss and wind chill (use blankets and insulating equipment)
• Maintain horizontal position
• Avoid rough movement and excess activity
• Monitor core temperature
• Monitor cardiac rhythm*
Assess responsiveness, breathing, and pulse
Pulse/ breathing present
Pulse/ breathing absent
What is core temperature?
34°C-36°C (mild hypothermia)
• Passive rewarming
• Active external rewarming
30°C-34°C (moderate hypothermia)
• Passive rewarming
• Active external rewarming of truncal areas only†‡
<30°C (severe hypothermia)
• Active internal rewarming sequence (below)
• Start CPR
• Defibrillate VF/VT up to a total of 3 shocks (200 J, 300 J, 360 J)
• Intubate
• Ventilate with warm, humid oxygen (42°C-46°C)†
• Establish IV
• Infuse warm normal saline (43°C)†
What is core temperature?
<30°C
≥30°C
• Continue CPR
• Withhold IV medications
• Limit shocks for VF/VT to 3 maximum
• Transport to hospital
• Continue CPR
• Give IV medications as indicated (but at longer than standard intervals)
• Repeat defibrillation for VF/VT as core temperature rises
Active internal rewarming†
• Warm IV fluid (43°C)
• Warm, humid oxygen (42°C-46°C)
• Peritoneal lavage (KCl-free fluid)
• Extracorporeal rewarming
• Esophageal rewarming tubes§
Continue active internal rewarming until:
• Core temperature ≥35°C or
• Return of spontaneous circulation or
• Resuscitative efforts cease

* This may require needle electrodes through the skin.
† Many experts think these interventions should be done only in-hospital though practices vary.
‡ Methods include electric or charcoal warming devices, hot water bottles, heating pads, radiant heat sources, and warming beds.
§ Esophageal rewarming tubes are widely used internationally and should become available in the United States.

Fig. 11. Algorithm for treatment of hypothermia. (From Emergency Cardiac Care Committee and Subcommittees, American Heart Association, American Heart Association. Guidelines for Cardiopulmonary Resuscitation and Emergency Cardiac Care. JAMA 268(16): 2171–2195, 1992. Copyright 1992, American Medical Association.)

Neurological Scoring Systems

Glasgow Coma Scale

Eye opening			
Spontaneous	4 points		
To speech	3		
To pain	2	☐	Patient's Score
None	1		
Best motor response			
Obeys commands	6 points		
Localizes	5		
Withdraws	4		
Abnormal flexion	3		
Extends	2	☐	Patient's Score
None	1		
Best verbal response			
Oriented	5 points		
Confused conversation	4		
Inappropriate words	3		
Incomprehensible sounds	2	☐	Patient's Score
None	1		
Total Glasgow Coma Scale Score Best Score: 15 Worst Score: 3		☐	

From Marino PL: *The ICU Book*. Malvern, PA, Lea & Febiger, 1991.

Pittsburgh Brain Stem Score

Designed to complement the Glasgow Coma Scale for the evaluation of nontraumatic injury. Includes an evaluation of brainstem reflexes. This score is added to the Glasgow score, as shown below. At present, there is only limited clinical experience with the combined scale.

Gag or cough reflex	Present = 2 Absent = 1	☐	
Lash reflex (either side)	Present = 2 Absent = 1	☐	
Corneal reflex (either side)	Present = 2 Absent = 1	☐	
Doll's eye or cold caloric reflex	Present = 2 Absent = 1	☐	
Right pupillary light reflex	Present = 2 Absent = 1	☐	
Left pupillary light reflex	Present = 2 Absent = 1	☐	
	PBSS	☐	(Best = 15) (Worst = 6)
	Add GCS	☐	(Best = 15) (Worst = 3)
	Combined Score	☐	(Best = 30) (Worst = 9)

From Safar P, Bircher NG: *Cardiopulmonary Cerebral Resuscitation,* 3rd ed. Philadelphia, WB Saunders, 1988, p. 262.

Acute Physiology And Chronic Health Evaluation

The APACHE II scoring system is used to rank the severity of illness in individual patients in a medical or surgical ICU. This scoring system does *not* apply to burn patients or to postoperative coronary artery bypass graft (CABG) patients.

The graph below is from a multicenter study of 515 ICU patients.* Only postoperative patients are included in this graph, but the medical patients showed a similar pattern.

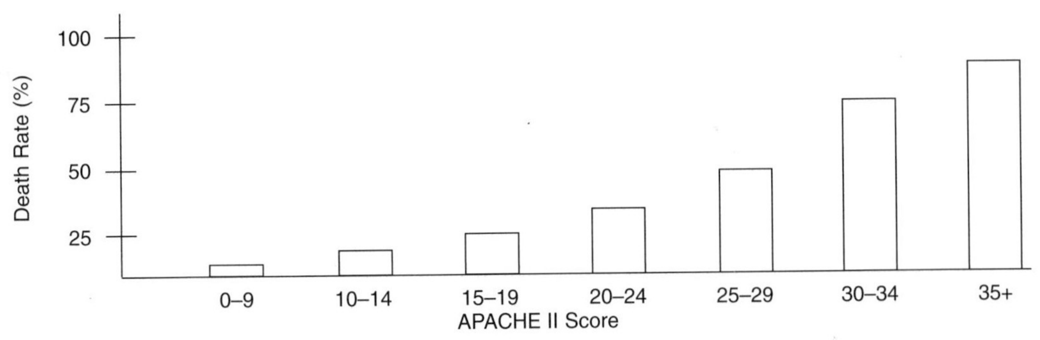

*Redrawn from Knaus WA, et al. APACHE II: A severity of disease classification system. Crit Care Med 13:818–829, 1985.

The APACHE II score is generated in 3 parts.

1. *Acute Physiology Score.* This consists of 12 measurements obtained within the first 24 hours of admission to the ICU. The most abnormal measurement for each variable is selected and the total APS is the sum of the scores from the individual measurements. The only nonobjective measure in this section is the Glascow Coma Score (GCS). The scoring method for the GCS is included.
2. *Age Adjustment.* A point total of zero to 6 points is alloted for the age of the patient.
3. *Chronic Health Adjustment.* Up to 5 additional points are allotted for chronic illnesses involving the major organ systems.

The final APACHE II score is the sum of the above 3 scores. The following is a list of the criteria used to generate scores in each part of the APACHE II scoring system.

From Marino PL: *The ICU Book.* Malvern, PA, Lea & Febiger, 1991.

Apache II (continued)

1. Acute Physiology Score

Variable	+4	+3	+2	+1	0	+1	+2	+3	+4
Temperature (°C)	≥41	39–40.9		38.5–38.9	36–38.4	34–35.9	32–33.9	30–31.9	≤29.9
Mean arterial BP	≥160	130–159	110–129		70–109		50–69		≤49
Heart rate	≥180	140–179	110–139		70–109		55–69	40–54	≤39
Respiratory rate	≥50	35–49		25–34	12–24	10–11	6–9		≤5
A-aPo_2* PaO_2†	≥500	350–499	200–349		<200 >70	61–70		55–60	<55
Arterial pH Serum HCO_3^{-}‡	≥7.7 ≥52	7.6–7.69 41–51.9		7.5–7.59 32–40.9	7.33–7.49 22–31.9		7.25–7.32 18–21.9	7.15–7.24 15–17.9	<7.15 <15
Serum Na^+	≥180	160–179	155–159	150–154	130–149		120–129	111–119	≤110
Serum K^+	≥7	6–6.9		5.5–5.9	3.5–5.4	3–3.4	2.5–2.9		<2.5
Serum creatinine	≥3.5	2–3.4	1.5–1.9		0.6–1.4		<0.6		

Hematocrit	≥60		50–59.9	46–49.9	30–45.9		20–29.9		<20
WBC count	≥40		20–39.9	15–19.9	3–14.9		1–2.9		<1
Glasgow Coma Score (GCS)[§]									
Acute Physiology Score (APS)									

*If FIO_2 > 50%
†If FIO_2 < 50%
‡Use only if no arterial blood gases
§Score = 15 − actual GCS

From Marino PL: *The ICU Book*. Malvern, PA, Lea & Febiger, 1991.

2. Age Adjustment

Age (Yrs)	Points
<44	0
45–54	2
55–64	3
65–74	5
>75	6

Apache II (continued)

3. Chronic Health Adjustment

Points can be added if the patient has a history of the following:

1. Biopsy-proven cirrhosis
2. New York Heart Association Class IV
3. Severe COPD (e.g., hypercapnia, home O_2, pulmonary hypertension)
4. Chronic dialysis
5. Immune compromise

If any of above are present, *add:* 2 points for elective surgery or for nonsurgical patients, 5 points for emergency surgery.

Apache II Score

1. ☐ APS ____________
2. ☐ Age Score ____________
3. ☐ Illness Score ____________

Total APACHE II ____________

From Marino PL: *The ICU Book.* Malvern, PA, Lea & Febiger, 1991.

Notice

The information and statements contained herein were obtained from the manufacturer or retailer of drugs or from recently published data and literature, including the following resources: *Physicians' Desk Reference, Facts and Comparisons,* the *American Hospital Formulary Service, Drug Dex,* and the manufacturers' drug inserts.

Extraordinary efforts have been made by the authors and the publisher of these cards to ensure that dosage recommendations are precise and in agreement with standards officially accepted at the time of publication.

It does happen, however, that dosage schedules are changed from time to time in light of accumulating clinical experience and continuing laboratory studies. This is most likely to occur in the case of recently introduced products.

It is urged that you always check the manufacturer's recommendations for dosage for the most current information.

BSA Nomogram

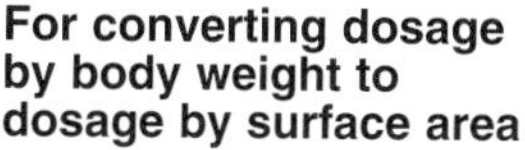

For converting dosage by body weight to dosage by surface area

A line connecting the height with the weight intersects the middle line at the corresponding surface area.

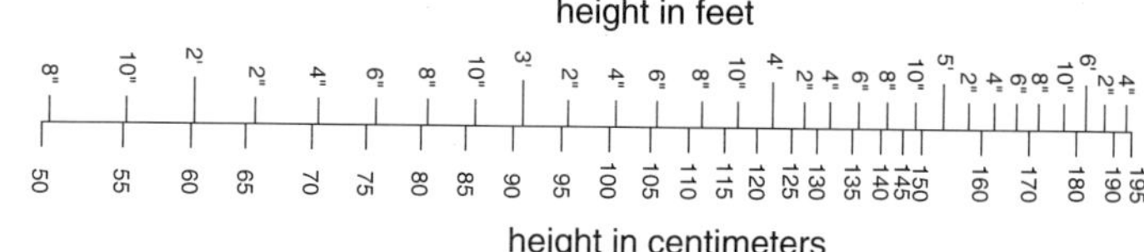

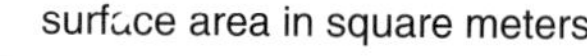

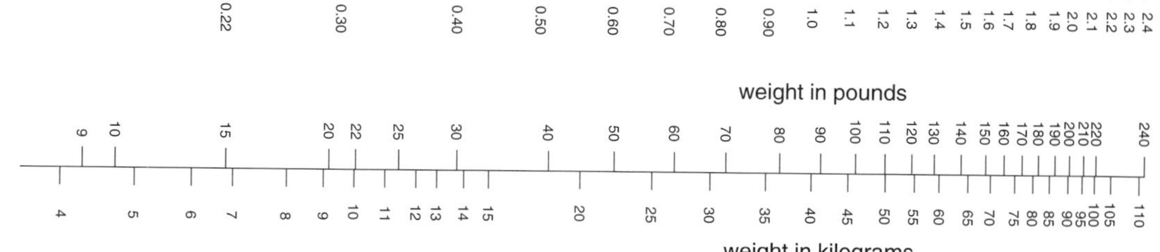

INTRAVENOUS MEDICATIONS FOR
CRITICAL CARE

Adenosine (Adenocard)

Pharmacology

Endogenous nucleoside present in all body cells

Decreases conduction time through the atrioventricular node (negative dromotropic effect) and may convert atrioventricular node reentrant tachycardia to sinus rhythm even in the setting of Wolff-Parkinson-White syndrome

May decrease blood pressure and peripheral vascular resistance, especially with large doses

Metabolism not affected by renal or hepatic failure

Indications

Conversion of paroxysmal supraventricular tachycardia to normal sinus rhythm, including those associated with Wolff-Parkinson-White bypass tracts

Unlabeled Use. Diagnostic stress testing in patients with suspected coronary artery disease

Administrative Guidelines

Administer via large vein, if possible, and follow with rapid saline flush

Do not repeat bolus doses if transient high-grade block develops

Contraindicated in patients with second- or third-degree block or sick sinus syndrome unless a functioning artificial pacemaker is present and in those with known hypersensitivity

Use with caution in those with first-degree block, in those with asthma, in the presence of carbamazepine, or during pregnancy

Overdosage should be managed by correction of specific adverse effects. These are usually self-limiting owing to the short half-life. Consider antagonism by methylxanthines including theophylline

Pharmacokinetics

Onset of Action. Immediate

Peak Effects. Within 10 seconds

Duration of Action. Approximately 10 seconds

IV (Distribution) Half-Life. Less than 10 seconds

Metabolism. Via red blood cells and vascular endothelial cells to inosine and AMP

Adenosine (Adenocard)

Dosing Information

Initial IV Bolus Dose for Dysrhythmias. 6 mg IV over 1–2 seconds

Subsequent Bolus Dosing. 12 mg if initial bolus is not effective after 1–2 minutes observation. May repeat 12-mg bolus dose a second time after additional 1–2 minutes

Maximum IV Bolus Dose. 12 mg per IV bolus; 30 mg cumulative dose

Infusion Dose for Diagnostic Stress Testing. 50 μg/kg/min initially, 140 μg/kg/min maximum

How Supplied

3 mg/mL—2-mL vials of 6 mg

Potential Drug Interactions

Potentiation of Adenosine Effects. Dipyridamole and carbamazepine

Antagonism of Adenosine Effects. Caffeine, theophylline, other methylxanthines

Principal Adverse Effects

CNS. Lightheadedness, blurred vision, dizziness, tingling in arms, numbness, apprehension, burning sensation, back pain, neck and arm heaviness, headache

Pulmonary. Dyspnea, hyperventilation, shortness of breath

CV. Flushing, palpitations, chest pain, hypotension, bradydysrhythmias, tachydysrythmias, heart block

GI. Nausea, metallic taste, throat tightness, groin pressure sensation

Adenosine (Adenocard)

Aminocaproic Acid (Amicar)

Pharmacology

Enhances hemostasis by inhibiting fibrinolysin (plasmin) and activation of profibrinolysin (plasminogen) by streptokinase in plasma

Indications

Management of life-threatening bleeding disorders secondary to systemic hyperfibrinolysis or urinary fibrinolysis

Unlabeled Uses. Amegakaryocytic thrombocytopenia, prevention of attacks of hereditary angioneurotic edema, traumatic hyphema, bleeding associated with thrombolytic agents and acute promyelocytic leukemia, prophylaxis against recurrent subarachnoid hemorrhage

Administrative Guidelines

Administer infusion via precision control device

Monitor coagulation studies and serum K^+ during administration (Amicar may elevate serum K^+)

Must have laboratory confirmation of hyperfibrinolysis before use—do not administer in the presence of disseminated intravascular coagulation without concomitant heparin therapy

Always dilute before venous infusion

Avoid rapid bolus administration to prevent hypotension, bradycardia, and dysrhythmias—infuse loading dose over 1 hour

Monitor serum CK during use and discontinue if a rise in CK is noted

Contraindicated with any intravascular clotting process, disseminated intravascular coagulation, upper urinary tract bleeding disorders, or known hypersensitivity

(continued below)

Pharmacokinetics

Onset of Action. Variable (1–3 hours)

Peak Effects. Variable (1–3 hours)

Duration of Action. 3–5 hours

Plasma (Distribution) Half-Life. 1–2 hours

Tissue (Elimination) Half-Life. 5 hours

Metabolism. No significant in vivo metabolism with 40–65% excreted unchanged in urine

Use with caution in patients with renal, hepatic, or cardiac disease

Overdosage has not been carefully described and no known antidote is reported by the manufacturer. The drug is removed by hemodialysis and peritoneal dialysis

Aminocaproic Acid (Amicar)

Dosing Information

Initial Infusion Rate. 4–5 g in 250 mL diluent over first hour

Maintenance Infusion Range. 1.0–1.25 g/hr in 50 mL diluent

Maximum Infusion Rate. 1.0–1.25 g/hr

Maximum Dose. 30 g over 24 hours total dose

Therapeutic Level

130 μg/mL

How Supplied

250 mg/mL—20-mL vials of 5 g
96-mL pharmacy bulk package of 24 g

Potential Drug Interactions

Potentiation of Clotting. Oral contraceptives or estrogen

Principal Adverse Effects

CNS. Dizziness, headache, tinnitus, weakness, delirium, hallucinations, psychotic reactions, convulsions, malaise, myopathy

CV. Hypotension, bradycardia, arrhythmias

GI. Nausea, cramps, diarrhea

Renal. Myoglobinuria and renal failure (secondary to rhabdomyolysis)

Miscellaneous. Rhabdomyolysis, skin rash, thrombophlebitis, prolongation of menstruation, nasal stuffiness, dry ejaculation

Aminocaproic Acid (Amicar) 15 g in 250 mL

■ Infusion Rate in mL/hr (pump setting) ■ Drug Dose in g/hr

mL/hr	g/hr	mL/hr	g/hr	mL/hr	g/hr	mL/hr	g/hr	mL/hr	g/hr	mL/hr	g/hr
1	0.06	21	1.26	41	2.46	61	3.66	81	4.86	101	6.06
2	0.12	22	1.32	42	2.52	62	3.72	82	4.92	102	6.12
3	0.18	23	1.38	43	2.58	63	3.78	83	4.98	103	6.18
4	0.24	24	1.44	44	2.64	64	3.84	84	5.04	104	6.24
5	0.30	25	1.50	45	2.70	65	3.90	85	5.10	105	6.30
6	0.36	26	1.56	46	2.76	66	3.96	86	5.16	106	6.36
7	0.42	27	1.62	47	2.82	67	4.02	87	5.22	107	6.42
8	0.48	28	1.68	48	2.88	68	4.08	88	5.28	108	6.48
9	0.54	29	1.74	49	2.94	69	4.14	89	5.34	109	6.54
10	0.60	30	1.80	50	3.00	70	4.20	90	5.40	110	6.60
11	0.66	31	1.86	51	3.06	71	4.26	91	5.46	111	6.66
12	0.72	32	1.92	52	3.12	72	4.32	92	5.52	112	6.72
13	0.78	33	1.98	53	3.18	73	4.38	93	5.58	113	6.78
14	0.84	34	2.04	54	3.24	74	4.44	94	5.64	114	6.84
15	0.90	35	2.10	55	3.30	75	4.50	95	5.70	115	6.90
16	0.96	36	2.16	56	3.36	76	4.56	96	5.76	116	6.96
17	1.02	37	2.22	57	3.42	77	4.62	97	5.82	117	7.02
18	1.08	38	2.28	58	3.48	78	4.68	98	5.88	118	7.08
19	1.14	39	2.34	59	3.54	79	4.74	99	5.94	119	7.14
20	1.20	40	2.40	60	3.60	80	4.80	100	6.00	120	7.20

Aminocaproic Acid (Amicar)

■ Infusion Rate in mL/hr (pump setting) ■ Drug Dose in g/hr

mL/hr	g/hr	mL/hr	g/hr	mL/hr	g/hr	mL/hr	g/hr	mL/hr	g/hr	mL/hr	g/hr
1	0.03	21	0.63	41	1.23	61	1.83	81	2.43	101	3.03
2	0.06	22	0.66	42	1.26	62	1.86	82	2.46	102	3.06
3	0.09	23	0.69	43	1.29	63	1.89	83	2.49	103	3.09
4	0.12	24	0.72	44	1.32	64	1.92	84	2.52	104	3.12
5	0.15	25	0.75	45	1.35	65	1.95	85	2.55	105	3.15
6	0.18	26	0.78	46	1.38	66	1.98	86	2.58	106	3.18
7	0.21	27	0.81	47	1.41	67	2.01	87	2.61	107	3.21
8	0.24	28	0.84	48	1.44	68	2.04	88	2.64	108	3.24
9	0.27	29	0.87	49	1.47	69	2.07	89	2.67	109	3.27
10	0.30	30	0.90	50	1.50	70	2.10	90	2.70	110	3.30
11	0.33	31	0.93	51	1.53	71	2.13	91	2.73	111	3.33
12	0.36	32	0.96	52	1.56	72	2.16	92	2.76	112	3.36
13	0.39	33	0.99	53	1.59	73	2.19	93	2.79	113	3.39
14	0.42	34	1.02	54	1.62	74	2.22	94	2.82	114	3.42
15	0.45	35	1.05	55	1.65	75	2.25	95	2.85	115	3.45
16	0.48	36	1.08	56	1.68	76	2.28	96	2.88	116	3.48
17	0.51	37	1.11	57	1.71	77	2.31	97	2.91	117	3.51
18	0.54	38	1.14	58	1.74	78	2.34	98	2.94	118	3.54
19	0.57	39	1.17	59	1.77	79	2.37	99	2.97	119	3.57
20	0.60	40	1.20	60	1.80	80	2.40	100	3.00	120	3.60

Amrinone Lactate (Inocor)

Pharmacology

Positive inotropic agent that may increase cellular levels of cyclic AMP (via phosphodiesterase inhibition)

Direct relaxant effect on vascular smooth muscle that decreases venous capacitance (preload) and arteriolar resistance (afterload)

Improves cardiac output and reduces pulmonary wedge pressure, left ventricular end diastolic pressure, systemic vascular resistance, and blood pressure

No significant effects on myocardial oxygen consumption

May induce tachydysrhythmias, especially in advanced heart failure patients

Indications

Short-term management of patients with congestive heart failure and depressed myocardial contractility who have not satisfactorily responded to digitalis, diuretics, or vasodilators

Unlabeled Use. Cardiotonic agent during advanced cardiac life support

Administrative Guidelines

Administer infusion via precision control device

Do not reconstitute with dextrose solutions (chemically incompatible)

Correct electrolyte abnormalities or hypovolemia, if possible, before use

Carefully monitor vital signs, ECG, platelet counts, electrolytes, renal chemistries, liver function tests, and, if possible, hemodynamics

Discontinue infusion if significant thrombocytopenia (<50,000) observed, significant hepatic dysfunction occurs, or gastrointestinal adverse effects noted

Contraindicated if hypersensitivity to amrinone or bisulfites present

Do not use with severe pulmonic or aortic stenosis, subaortic obstructive lesions, or in acute myocardial infarction

Use cautiously in those with hypovolemia or ventricular dysrhythmias

Overdosage is rare and may manifest as hypotension or significant dysrhythmias. Manage with discontinuation of infusion and general supportive measures

Pharmacokinetics

Onset of Action. 2–5 minutes

Peak Effects. Within 10 minutes

Duration of Action. 30 minutes–2 hours

IV Bolus (Distribution) Half-Life. 5 minutes

IV Infusion (Elimination) Half-Life. 4–6 hours but may be up to 13 hours with heart failure

Metabolism. Conjugated by liver with 10–40% excreted unchanged in urine at 24 hours

Amrinone Lactate (Inocor)

Dosing Information

Initial Loading Dose. 0.75 mg/kg IV bolus slowly over 2–3 minutes—may repeat initial bolus after 30 minutes

Maintenance Infusion Range. 5–10 μg/kg/min

Maximum Infusion Range. 10–20 μg/kg/min

Do not exceed 10 mg/kg total daily dose including boluses

Therapeutic Levels

0.5–7.0 μg/mL

Titration Guideline

Suggested Regimen. Adjust infusion by 2.5 μg/kg/min every 10 minutes as required

How Supplied

5 mg/mL—20-mL ampuls of 100 mg

Potential Drug Interactions

Potentiation of Inocor Effects. Digitalis, disopyramide

Principal Adverse Effects

CV. Arrhythmias, hypotension

GI. Nausea, vomiting, abdominal pain, anorexia, and hepatic enzyme elevation

Heme. Dose-dependent thrombocytopenia

Allergic. Hypersensitivity reactions

Miscellaneous. Fever, chest pain, burning at infusion site

Amrinone Lactate (Inocor) 500 mg in 500 mL

DRUG DOSE in μg/kg/min

Patient's Weight

kg / lbs	40 / 88	45 / 99	50 / 110	55 / 121	60 / 132	65 / 143	70 / 154	75 / 165	80 / 176	85 / 187	90 / 198	95 / 209	100 / 220	105 / 231	110 / 242
Infusion rate in mL/hr															
5	2.1	1.9	1.7	1.5	1.4	1.3	1.2	1.1	1.0	1.0	0.9	0.9	0.8	0.8	0.8
10	4.2	3.7	3.3	3.0	2.8	2.6	2.4	2.2	2.1	2.0	1.9	1.8	1.7	1.6	1.5
15	6.2	5.6	5.0	4.5	4.2	3.8	3.6	3.3	3.1	2.9	2.8	2.6	2.5	2.4	2.3
20	8.3	7.4	6.7	6.1	5.6	5.1	4.8	4.4	4.2	3.9	3.7	3.5	3.3	3.2	3.0
25	10.4	9.3	8.3	7.6	6.9	6.4	6.0	5.6	5.2	4.9	4.6	4.4	4.2	4.0	3.8
30	12.5	11.1	10.0	9.1	8.3	7.7	7.1	6.7	6.2	5.9	5.6	5.3	5.0	4.8	4.5
35	14.6	13.0	11.7	10.6	9.7	9.0	8.3	7.8	7.3	6.9	6.5	6.1	5.8	5.6	5.3
40	16.7	14.8	13.3	12.1	11.1	10.3	9.5	8.9	8.3	7.8	7.4	7.0	6.7	6.3	6.1
45	18.7	16.7	15.0	13.6	12.5	11.5	10.7	10.0	9.4	8.8	8.3	7.9	7.5	7.1	6.8
50	20.8	18.5	16.7	15.2	13.9	12.8	11.9	11.1	10.4	9.9	9.3	8.8	8.3	7.9	7.6
55	22.9	20.4	18.3	16.7	15.3	14.1	13.1	12.2	11.5	10.8	10.2	9.6	9.2	8.7	8.3
60	25.0	22.2	20.0	18.2	16.7	15.4	14.3	13.3	12.5	11.8	11.1	10.5	10.0	9.5	9.1
65	27.1	24.1	21.7	19.7	18.1	16.7	15.5	14.4	13.5	12.7	12.0	11.4	10.8	10.3	9.3
70	29.2	25.9	23.3	21.2	19.4	17.9	16.7	15.6	14.8	13.7	13.0	12.3	11.7	11.1	10.6
75	31.2	27.8	25.0	22.7	20.8	19.2	17.9	16.7	15.6	14.7	13.9	13.2	12.5	11.9	11.4
80	33.3	29.6	26.7	24.2	22.2	20.5	19.0	17.8	16.7	15.7	14.8	14.0	13.3	12.7	12.1
85	35.4	31.5	28.3	25.8	23.6	21.8	20.2	18.9	17.7	16.7	15.7	14.9	14.2	13.5	12.9
90	37.5	33.3	30.0	27.3	25.0	23.1	21.4	20.0	18.7	17.6	16.7	15.8	15.0	14.3	13.6
95	39.6	35.2	31.7	28.8	26.4	34.4	22.6	21.1	19.8	18.6	17.6	16.7	15.8	15.1	14.4
100	41.7	37.0	33.3	30.3	27.8	25.6	23.8	22.2	20.8	19.6	18.5	17.5	16.7	15.9	15.2
105	43.7	38.9	35.0	31.8	29.2	26.9	25.0	23.3	21.9	20.6	19.4	18.4	17.5	16.7	15.9
110	45.8	40.7	36.7	33.3	30.6	28.2	26.2	24.4	22.9	21.6	20.4	19.3	18.3	17.5	16.7
115	47.9	42.6	38.3	34.8	31.9	29.5	27.4	25.6	24.0	22.5	21.3	20.2	19.2	18.3	17.4
120	50.0	44.4	40.0	36.4	33.3	30.8	28.6	26.7	25.0	23.5	22.2	21.1	20.0	19.0	18.2

DRUG DOSE in μg/kg/min

Patient's Weight

Infusion rate in mL/hr	kg 40 / lbs 88	45 / 99	50 / 110	55 / 121	60 / 132	65 / 143	70 / 154	75 / 165	80 / 176	85 / 187	90 / 198	95 / 209	100 / 220	105 / 231	110 / 242
5	4.17	3.70	3.33	3.03	2.78	2.56	2.38	2.22	2.08	1.96	1.85	1.75	1.67	1.59	1.52
10	8.33	7.41	6.67	6.06	5.56	5.13	4.76	4.44	4.17	3.92	3.70	3.51	3.33	3.17	3.03
15	12.50	11.11	10.00	9.09	8.33	7.69	7.14	6.67	6.25	5.88	5.56	5.26	5.00	4.76	4.55
20	16.67	14.81	13.33	12.12	11.11	10.26	9.52	8.89	8.33	7.84	7.41	7.02	6.67	6.35	6.06
25	20.83	18.52	16.67	15.15	13.89	12.82	11.90	11.11	10.42	9.80	9.26	8.77	8.33	7.94	7.58
30	25.00	22.22	20.00	18.18	16.67	15.38	14.29	13.33	12.50	11.76	11.11	10.53	10.00	9.52	9.09
35	29.17	25.93	23.33	21.21	19.44	17.95	16.67	15.56	14.58	13.73	12.96	12.28	11.67	11.11	10.61
40	33.33	29.63	26.67	24.24	22.22	20.51	19.05	17.78	16.67	15.69	14.81	14.04	13.33	12.70	12.12
45	37.50	33.33	30.00	27.27	25.00	23.08	21.43	20.00	18.75	17.65	16.67	15.79	15.00	14.29	13.64
50	41.67	37.04	33.33	30.30	27.78	25.64	23.81	22.22	20.83	19.61	18.52	17.54	16.67	15.87	15.15
55	45.83	40.74	36.67	33.33	30.56	28.21	26.19	24.44	22.92	21.57	20.37	19.30	18.33	17.46	16.67
60	50.00	44.44	40.00	36.36	33.33	30.77	28.57	26.67	25.00	23.53	22.22	21.05	20.00	19.05	18.18
65	54.17	48.15	43.33	39.39	36.11	33.33	30.95	28.89	27.08	25.49	24.07	22.81	21.67	20.63	19.70
70	58.33	51.85	46.67	42.42	38.89	35.90	33.33	31.11	29.17	27.45	25.93	24.56	23.33	22.22	21.21
75	62.50	55.56	50.00	45.45	41.67	38.46	35.71	33.33	31.25	29.41	27.78	26.32	25.00	23.81	22.73
80	66.67	59.26	53.33	48.48	44.44	41.03	38.10	35.56	33.33	31.37	29.63	28.07	26.67	25.40	24.24
85	70.83	62.96	56.67	51.52	47.22	43.59	40.48	37.78	35.42	33.33	31.48	29.82	28.33	26.98	25.76
90	75.00	66.67	60.00	54.55	50.00	46.15	42.86	40.00	37.50	35.29	33.33	31.58	30.00	28.57	27.27
95	79.17	70.37	63.33	57.58	52.78	48.72	45.24	42.22	39.58	37.25	35.19	33.33	31.67	30.16	28.79
100	83.33	74.07	66.67	60.61	55.56	51.28	47.62	44.44	41.67	39.22	37.04	35.09	33.33	31.75	30.30
105	87.50	77.78	70.00	63.64	58.33	53.85	50.00	46.67	43.75	41.18	38.89	36.84	35.00	33.33	31.82
110	91.67	81.48	73.33	66.67	61.11	56.41	52.38	48.89	45.83	43.14	40.74	38.60	36.67	34.92	33.33
115	95.83	85.19	76.67	69.70	63.89	58.97	54.76	51.11	47.92	45.10	42.59	40.35	38.33	36.51	34.85
120	100.00	88.89	80.00	72.73	66.67	61.54	57.14	53.33	50.00	47.06	44.44	42.11	40.00	38.10	36.36

Anistreplase (APSAC, Eminase)

Pharmacology

Thrombolytic proenzyme consisting of inactive complex of streptokinase, human Lys-plasminogen, and an anisoyl group

Mechanism of action involves deacylation with formation of Lys-plasminogen activator complex, which converts plasminogen to plasmin. Thereafter, plasmin degrades fibrin, fibrinogen, and other procoagulant proteins

Site of action includes endogenous lysis by diffusion of activator complex into the thrombus and exogenous lysis of thrombus by circulating plasmin

Enhanced fibrin specificity compared with streptokinase

Indications

Lysis of coronary thrombi during acute evolving transmural myocardial infarction—initiate therapy preferably within **6** hours of symptom onset

Administrative Guidelines

Administer as soon as possible after symptom onset—efficacy may be time dependent

Continuously monitor ECG and carefully follow vital signs

When preparing infusion, do not add other medications to the vial and reconstitute with 5 mL of sterile water for injection USP. Gently tilt and roll vial but do not shake. Discard solution if highly colored, flocculation noted, or not administered within 30 minutes

Avoid intramuscular injections before, during, and 24 hours after anistreplase therapy. Do not attempt central venous access or arterial puncture during this period unless absolutely essential (upper extremity sites are preferred)

Minimize performance of venipuncture and handling of patient. Compress venipuncture sites for up to 30 minutes to control minor bleeding, apply a pressure dressing, and check site frequently

(continued below)

Pharmacokinetics

Onset of Action. Within 45 minutes

Peak Effects. Approximately 45 minutes–2 hours

Duration of Action. Approximately 4–6 hours

Fibrinolytic Activity Half-Life. 70 minutes–2 hours

Metabolism. Plasma deacylation of the activator complex

Apply local pressure to minor surface bleeding areas as necessary but do ***not*** alter the infusion dose with superficial bleeding

Effectiveness of anistreplase may be diminished if administered 5 days–6 months following prior anistreplase or streptokinase therapy or streptococcal infection (owing to elevated antistreptococcal antibody levels)

Efficacy and bleeding risk do not directly correlate with laboratory studies of the lytic state

The role of heparin in preventing recurrent thrombosis has not been established. Consider heparin infusion 4–8 hours after anistreplase administration

Contraindicated with known hypersensitivity, active internal bleeding, severe uncontrolled hypertension, history of cerebrovascular accident, established bleeding diathesis, intracranial neoplasm, aneurysm or arteriovenous malformation, and intracranial or intraspinal surgery or trauma within 2 months

Use with extreme caution in hypertension exceeding 180 mmHg systolic or 110 mmHg diastolic pressure

(continued on page 20)

and recent (within 10 days) serious trauma, major surgery, organ biopsy, gastrointestinal bleeding, obstetrical delivery, or puncture of a noncompressible artery

Use with caution following cardiopulmonary resuscitation, minor trauma within 10 days, suspected mural thrombus, during pregnancy, hemorrhagic diabetic retinopathy, cerebrovascular disease, acute pericarditis, subacute bacterial endocarditis, septic thrombophlebitis or occluded arteriovenous cannula at the site of serious infection, severe hepatic or renal disease, atrial fibrillation, conditions associated with increased bleeding risk, and in those over 75 years of age

Overdosage may manifest with severe hemorrhage. Provide general supportive measures and fluid resuscitate with volume expanders other than dextran. Transfuse with packed red blood cells, fresh frozen plasma and cryoprecipitate as needed. Although unproven, IV aminocaproic acid may be efficacious in life-threatening cases

Dosing Information

IV Bolus Dose. 30 units direct injection over 2–5 minutes

Maximum IV Bolus Dose. 30 units

How Supplied

30-unit vials—each unit contains approximately 36,000 IU of streptokinase

Potential Drug Interactions

Potentiation of Anistreplase Effects. Heparin, aspirin, dipyridamole, ticlopidine, oral anticoagulants

Antagonism of Anistreplase Effects. Aminocaproic acid

Principal Adverse Effects

CNS. Cerebrovascular hemorrhage, chills, fever, headache, agitation, paresthesias, tremor, vertigo

Pulmonary. Hemoptysis, dyspnea, bronchospasm, pulmonary edema

CV. Bradycardia, hypotension, reperfusion-related atrial and ventricular dysrhythmias, conduction disturbances, chest pain, cardiac rupture, shock, arterial emboli

GI. Nausea, vomiting, gingival or gastrointestinal bleeding, elevated liver function tests

Renal. Hematuria and proteinuria

Musculoskeletal. Myalgia, arthralgia

(continued on page 22)

Heme. Spontaneous superficial or internal hemorrhage, thrombocytopenia

Allergic. Anaphylactoid and anaphylactic reactions, delayed hypersensitivity responses including rash, urticaria, angioedema, pruritus

Miscellaneous. Hyperthermia

Atracurium Besylate (Tracrium)

Pharmacology

Synthetic nondepolarizing skeletal muscle relaxant that competitively blocks cholinergic receptor sites

May precipitate histamine release and hypotension, especially with doses of 0.5 mg/kg or greater

No significant direct cardiovascular effects or effects on consciousness, cerebration, or pain

Indications

Adjunctive therapy during intubation or general anesthesia; skeletal muscle relaxation during surgery or mechanical ventilation

Administrative Guidelines

Administer infusion via precision control device

Continuously monitor ECG, respiration, and vital signs

Always have anticholinesterase reversal agents, endotracheal intubation equipment, mechanical ventilation, and skilled personnel in attendance

Do not use with lactated Ringer's USP (degrades more readily)

Dilute with 5% dextrose injection USP or 0.9% sodium chloride injection USP

Do not administer with alkaline solutions, especially barbiturates (atracurium may be inactivated)

Inspect solution for discoloration or particulate matter and discard if evident

Do not administer by intramuscular injection

Safety has not been established in pregnancy, children less than 1 month old, and those with bronchial asthma

(continued below)

Pharmacokinetics

Onset of Action. 2–3 minutes

Peak Effects. 3–10 minutes

Duration of Action. 20–35 minutes before recovery begins—60–70 minutes for 95% recovery without reversal

IV Bolus (Distribution) Half-Life. 2–3 minutes

IV Infusion (Elimination) Half-Life. Approximately 20 minutes

Metabolism. Via Hoffman elimination and enzymatic ester hydrolysis. Increased temperature and pH enhance metabolism

Carefully monitor adductor pollicis muscle with twitch response to peripheral nerve stimulation during use

Allow patients to recover from succinylcholine before use

May induce malignant hyperthermia

Tachyphylaxis may develop with prolonged use in the intensive care unit

Increased dose may be required in burn patients who develop tachyphylaxis

Dose reduction is not required with renal or hepatic disease

Use only ***after*** unconsciousness produced and adequate general anesthesia applied

Contraindicated with known hypersensitivity

Use with caution in patients with history of allergic responses in whom histamine release may be harmful, bradycardic individuals, those with severe electrolyte abnormalities, diffuse carcinomatosis, neuromuscular disease such as myasthenia gravis, and nursing mothers

(continued on page 26)

Atracurium Besylate (Tracrium)

Overdosage may potentiate pharmacologic effects, including histamine release, hypotension, respiratory depression, and neuromuscular blockade. Manage with appropriate fluids, cardiopulmonary support, and mechanical ventilation. Consider anticholinesterase agents such as neostigmine and anticholinergic drugs such as atropine. There is no established role for dialysis

Dosing Information

Initial Loading Dose. 200–500 μg/kg over 1 minute

Maintenance Dose. 80–100 μg/kg (every 15–45 minutes as necessary)

Initial Infusion Rate. 9–10 μg/kg/min

Maintenance Infusion Rate. 2–15 μg/kg/min

Maximum Infusion Rate. 15 μg/kg/min

Titration Guideline

Suggested Regimen. Adjust infusion by 1–2 μg/kg/min as necessary for neuromuscular blockade

How Supplied

10 mg/mL—5-mL vials and ampuls of 50 mg
10-mL multidose vials of 100 mg

Potential Drug Interactions

Potentiation of Atracurium Effects. Acidosis, enflurane, isoflurane, halothane, cholinergic and cholinesterase drugs, aminoglycosides, polymyxins, lithium, magnesium salts, procainamide, quinidine, succinylcholine

Antagonism of Atracurium Effects. Alkalosis, lactated Ringer's injection USP, anticholinesterase, and anticholinergic agents

Principal Adverse Effects

CV. Hypotension, tachycardia, bradycardia, flushing

Pulmonary. Laryngospasm, dyspnea, bronchospasm

Musculoskeletal. Inadequate relaxation, prolonged blockade

Dermatological. Urticaria, rash, injection site reaction

Allergic. Anaphylactic and other histamine-mediated responses

Atracurium Besylate (Tracrium) 50 mg in 100 mL

DRUG DOSE in µg/kg/min

Patient's Weight

Infusion Rate in mL/hr	kg/lbs 40/88	45/99	50/110	55/121	60/132	65/143	70/154	75/165	80/176	85/187	90/198	95/209	100/220	105/231	110/242
5	1.04	0.93	0.83	0.76	0.69	0.64	0.60	0.56	0.52	0.49	0.46	0.44	0.42	0.40	0.38
10	2.08	1.85	1.67	1.52	1.39	1.28	1.19	1.11	1.04	0.98	0.93	0.88	0.83	0.79	0.76
15	3.13	2.78	2.50	2.27	2.08	1.92	1.79	1.67	1.56	1.47	1.39	1.32	1.25	1.19	1.14
20	4.17	3.70	3.33	3.03	2.78	2.56	2.38	2.22	2.08	1.96	1.85	1.75	1.67	1.59	1.52
25	5.21	4.63	4.17	3.79	3.47	3.21	2.98	2.78	2.60	2.45	2.31	2.19	2.08	1.98	1.89
30	6.25	5.56	5.00	4.55	4.17	3.85	3.57	3.33	3.13	2.94	2.78	2.63	2.50	2.38	2.27
35	7.29	6.48	5.83	5.30	4.86	4.49	4.17	3.89	3.65	3.43	3.24	3.07	2.92	2.78	2.65
40	8.33	7.41	6.67	6.06	5.56	5.13	4.76	4.44	4.17	3.92	3.70	3.51	3.33	3.17	3.03
45	9.38	8.33	7.50	6.82	6.25	5.77	5.36	5.00	4.69	4.41	4.17	3.95	3.75	3.57	3.41
50	10.42	9.26	8.33	7.58	6.94	6.41	5.95	5.56	5.21	4.90	4.63	4.39	4.17	3.97	3.79
55	11.46	10.19	9.17	8.33	7.64	7.05	6.55	6.11	5.73	5.39	5.09	4.82	4.58	4.37	4.17
60	12.50	11.11	10.00	9.09	8.33	7.69	7.14	6.67	6.25	5.88	5.56	5.26	5.00	4.76	4.55
65	13.54	12.04	10.83	9.85	9.03	8.33	7.74	7.22	6.77	6.37	6.02	5.70	5.42	5.16	4.92
70	14.58	12.96	11.67	10.61	9.72	8.97	8.33	7.78	7.29	6.86	6.48	6.14	5.83	5.56	5.30
75	15.63	13.89	12.50	11.36	10.42	9.62	8.93	8.33	7.81	7.35	6.94	6.58	6.25	5.95	5.68
80	16.67	14.81	13.33	12.12	11.11	10.26	9.52	8.89	8.33	7.84	7.41	7.02	6.67	6.35	6.06
85	17.71	15.74	14.17	12.88	11.81	10.90	10.12	9.44	8.85	8.33	7.87	7.46	7.08	6.75	6.44
90	18.75	16.67	15.00	13.64	12.50	11.54	10.71	10.00	9.38	8.82	8.33	7.89	7.50	7.14	6.82
95	19.79	17.59	15.83	14.39	13.19	12.18	11.31	10.56	9.90	9.31	8.80	8.33	7.92	7.54	7.20
100	20.83	18.52	16.67	15.15	13.89	12.82	11.90	11.11	10.42	9.80	9.26	8.77	8.33	7.94	7.58
105	21.88	19.44	17.50	15.91	14.58	13.46	12.50	11.67	10.94	10.29	9.72	9.21	8.75	8.33	7.95
110	22.92	20.37	18.33	16.67	15.28	14.10	13.10	12.22	11.46	10.78	10.19	9.65	9.17	8.73	8.33
115	23.96	21.30	19.17	17.42	15.97	14.74	13.69	12.78	11.98	11.27	10.65	10.09	9.58	9.13	8.71
120	25.00	22.22	20.00	18.18	16.67	15.38	14.29	13.33	12.50	11.76	11.11	10.53	10.00	9.52	[illegible]

DRUG DOSE in μg/kg/min

Patient's weight

Infusion Rate in mL/hr	kg 40 / lbs 88	kg 45 / lbs 99	kg 50 / lbs 110	kg 55 / lbs 121	kg 60 / lbs 132	kg 65 / lbs 143	kg 70 / lbs 154	kg 75 / lbs 165	kg 80 / lbs 176	kg 85 / lbs 187	kg 90 / lbs 198	kg 95 / lbs 209	kg 100 / lbs 220	kg 105 / lbs 231	kg 110 / lbs 242
5	2.08	1.85	1.67	1.52	1.39	1.28	1.19	1.11	1.04	0.98	0.93	0.88	0.83	0.79	0.76
10	4.17	3.70	3.33	3.03	2.78	2.56	2.38	2.22	2.08	1.96	1.85	1.75	1.67	1.59	1.52
15	6.25	5.56	5.00	4.55	4.17	3.85	3.57	3.33	3.13	2.94	2.78	2.63	2.50	2.38	2.27
20	8.33	7.41	6.67	6.06	5.56	5.13	4.76	4.44	4.17	3.92	3.70	3.51	3.33	3.17	3.03
25	10.42	9.26	8.33	7.58	6.94	6.41	5.95	5.56	5.21	4.90	4.63	4.39	4.17	3.97	3.79
30	12.50	11.11	10.00	9.09	8.33	7.69	7.14	6.67	6.25	5.88	5.56	5.26	5.00	4.76	4.55
35	14.58	12.96	11.67	10.61	9.72	8.97	8.33	7.78	7.29	6.86	6.48	6.14	5.83	5.56	5.30
40	16.67	14.81	13.33	12.12	11.11	10.26	9.52	8.89	8.33	7.84	7.41	7.02	6.67	6.35	6.06
45	18.75	16.67	15.00	13.64	12.50	11.54	10.71	10.00	9.38	8.82	8.33	7.89	7.50	7.14	6.82
50	20.83	18.52	16.67	15.15	13.89	12.82	11.90	11.11	10.42	9.80	9.26	8.77	8.33	7.94	7.58
55	22.92	20.37	18.33	16.67	15.28	14.10	13.10	12.22	11.46	10.78	10.19	9.65	9.17	8.73	8.33
60	25.00	22.22	20.00	18.18	16.67	15.38	14.29	13.33	12.50	11.76	11.11	10.53	10.00	9.52	9.09
65	27.08	24.07	21.67	19.70	18.06	16.67	15.48	14.44	13.54	12.75	12.04	11.40	10.83	10.32	9.85
70	29.17	25.93	23.33	21.21	19.44	17.95	16.67	15.56	14.58	13.73	12.96	12.28	11.67	11.11	10.61
75	31.25	27.78	25.00	22.73	20.83	19.23	17.86	16.67	15.63	14.71	13.89	13.16	12.50	11.90	11.36
80	33.33	29.63	26.67	24.24	22.22	20.51	19.05	17.78	16.67	15.69	14.81	14.04	13.33	12.70	12.12
85	35.42	31.48	28.33	25.76	23.61	21.79	20.24	18.89	17.71	16.67	15.74	14.91	14.17	13.49	12.88
90	37.50	33.33	30.00	27.27	25.00	23.08	21.43	20.00	18.75	17.65	16.67	15.79	15.00	14.29	13.64
95	39.58	35.19	31.67	28.79	26.39	24.36	22.62	21.11	19.79	18.63	17.59	16.67	15.83	15.08	14.39
100	41.67	37.04	33.33	30.30	27.78	25.64	23.81	22.22	20.83	19.61	18.52	17.54	16.67	15.87	15.15
105	43.75	38.89	35.00	31.82	29.17	26.92	25.00	23.33	21.88	20.59	19.44	18.42	17.50	16.67	15.91
110	45.83	40.74	36.67	33.33	30.56	28.21	26.19	24.44	22.92	21.57	20.37	19.30	18.33	17.46	16.67
115	47.92	42.59	38.33	34.85	31.94	29.49	27.38	25.56	23.96	22.55	21.30	20.18	19.17	18.25	17.42
120	50.00	44.44	40.00	36.36	33.33	30.77	28.57	26.67	25.00	23.53	22.22	21.05	20.00	19.05	18.18

Atropine Sulfate

Pharmacology

Naturally occurring anticholinergic and antimuscarinic agent. Competitively inhibits acetylcholine effects (parasympathetic inhibition) but does not prevent acetylcholine's release

Typically produces stimulant effects on CNS manifesting as moderate respiratory stimulation and mild vagal excitation

Stimulant action on heart may abolish bradycardia and atrioventricular block

Inhibits secretion of sweat, bronchial, and salivary glands

Inhibits contractions of uterus and bladder and reduces gastrointestinal tract motility

Potent bronchodilator

May dilate pupils (mydriasis), paralyze accommodation of pupils (cycloplegia), and increase intraocular pressure

Administrative Guidelines

Carefully monitor ECG and vital signs

Do not use less than 0.4-mg doses as smaller doses may produce dose-dependent vagal stimulating response (paradoxic effect)

Do not admix with norepinephrine, metaraminol, methohexital, or sodium bicarbonate

May be administered via endotracheal tube

Contraindicated in patients with known hypersensitivity, tachycardia secondary to thyrotoxicosis or heart failure, narrow-angle glaucoma, adhesions between the iris and lens, obstructive uropathy, myasthenia gravis, acute hemorrhagic states associated with cardiovascular instability, gastrointestinal obstructions or hypomotility disorders, and severe ulcerative colitis

Use with caution in febrile patients or those exposed to increased ambient temperature (may precipitate hyperthermic crisis)

(continued below)

Indications

Reduction of salivary, nasal, and respiratory secretions during anesthesia

Prevention of cholinergic effects during surgery including bradycardia, hypotension, and cardiac dysrhythmias

Management of hypermotility disorders of the gastrointestinal and genitourinary tracts

Adjunctive therapy of biliary and ureteral colic and peptic ulcer disease

Relaxation of the colon and gastrointestinal tract during hypotonic duodenography

Diagnosis and management of sinus node dysfunction including carotid sinus hypersensitivity

Prevention and treatment of symptomatic bradycardia, hypotension, and vagally mediated atrioventricular block, especially during advanced cardiac life support

Anticholinesterase poisonings due to certain mushroom species (Amanita muscaria), organophosphorus insecticides, or excessive cholinergic medications

Cautiously administer to patients over 40 years of age, individuals requiring mental alertness and preserved visual acuity, those with hyperthyroidism, hepatic or renal dysfunction, autonomic neuropathy, congestive heart failure, ischemic heart disease, tachydysrhythmias, debilitated patients with chronic pulmonary disease, hypertension, gastrointestinal infections, diarrhea or ulcerative colitis, patients on digitalis glycosides, cholinergics, or neostigmine, those with asthma and allergies, biliary tract disease, gastric ulcer disease, prostatic hypertrophy or partial obstructive uropathy, hiatal hernia with reflux, and brain damage or spastic states

Overdosage may manifest with CNS disturbances, including delirium, coma, and acute psychotic behavior; fever, circulatory failure with tachycardia; gastrointestinal disturbances; urinary urgency; and visual disturbances with mydriasis. Provide supportive measures and consider neostigmine methylsulfate 0.5–2.0 mg IV with repeat doses as needed. The role of physostigmine salicylate is unclear and should be

(continued on page 32)

Atropine Sulfate

Pharmacokinetics

Onset of Action. Within 2 minutes

Peak Effects. Within 2–4 minutes

Duration of Action. Less than 45 minutes

Plasma Half-Life. Approximately 2–3 hours

Metabolism. Via liver with 30–50% excreted in urine as unchanged drug

reserved for life-threatening emergencies. Use 2 mg slow IV push initially, then 1–2 mg IV every 20 minutes as necessary to reverse muscarinic effects. Thereafter, 1–4 mg IV every 30–60 minutes may be used. There is no established role for dialysis

Dosing Information

Bradycardia and Heart Block During CPR. 0.5–1.0 mg IV push. May repeat at 3–5 minute intervals as necessary up to 0.04 mg/kg. Shorter dosing intervals in extreme situations may be helpful

Ventricular Asystole. 1.0 mg IV push. May repeat at 3–5 minute intervals as necessary up to 0.04 mg/kg. Shorter dosing intervals in extreme situations may be helpful

Muscarinic Blockade of Anticholinesterase Agents. 0.6–1.2 mg IV for each 0.5–2.5 mg neostigmine methylsulfate or 10–20 mg pyridostigmine dose administered (inject atropine a few minutes before the anticholinesterase agent is given)

Organophosphorus Poisonings. 1–2 mg IV push. May repeat every 5–60 minutes as necessary. In severe cases, 2–6 mg IV initially. Repeat at 5–60 minute intervals as required up to approximately 50 mg over 24 hours

Antidote to Mushroom Poisoning. 1–2 mg IV every hour until respiratory symptoms dissipate

(continued on page 34)

Potential Drug Interactions

Potentiation of Atropine Effects. Tricyclic antidepressants, benzodiazepines, antiparkinson drugs, antihistamines, antipsychotics, nitrates, nitrites, alkalinizing agents, alphaprodine, buclizine, orphenadrine, primidone, thioxanthenes, corticosteroids, haloperidol, disopyramide, procainamide, quinidine, amantadine, glutethimide

Antagonism of Atropine Effects. Guanethidine, reserpine, and histamine (all enhance gastric acid secretion)

Possibly Potentiated by Atropine. Sympathomimetics, cyclopropane, nitrofurantoin, thiazides

Possibly Antagonized by Atropine. Metoclopramide.

Atropine may delay or alter absorption of ketoconazole, acetaminophen, and levodopa

Atropine Sulfate

Antidote to Cholinesterase Inhibitors. 2–4 mg IV push. May repeat every 5–10 minutes as required or until atropine toxicity evident

Other Uses. 0.4–0.6 mg IV push. May repeat at 5-minute intervals as necessary

How Supplied

0.1 mg/mL—syringes of 5 mL (0.5 mg) and 10 mL (1.0 mg)

0.3 mg/mL—vials of 1 mL (0.3 mg) and 30 mL (9.0 mg)

0.4 mg/mL—ampuls of 1 mL (0.4 mg)
vials of 1 mL (0.4 mg), 20 mL (8.0 mg), and 30 mL (12 mg)

0.5 mg/mL—vials of 1 mL (0.5 mg) and 30 mL (15 mg)
syringes of 5 mL (2.5 mg)

0.8 mg/mL—ampuls of 0.5 mL (0.4 mg) and 1 mL (0.8 mg) syringes of 0.5 mL (0.4 mg)

1 mg/mL—ampuls of 1 mL (1.0 mg)
vials of 1 mL (1.0 mg)
syringes of 10 mL (10 mg)

Principal Adverse Effects

CNS. Restlessness, hallucinations, delirium, coma, headache, weakness, fever, insomnia, excitement, depression, anxiety, confusion, psychotic behavior, altered moods, dysarthria, agitation, abnormal gait and motor activity, ataxia, tremor, dizziness

Pulmonary. Tachypnea, respiratory paralysis

CV. Palpitations, tachydysrhythmias, hypertension, bradycardia, circulatory collapse in severe cases

GI. Nausea, vomiting, dry mouth, constipation, dysphagia, ileus, gastroesophageal reflux, heartburn

GU. Impaired micturition, urinary retention, impotence

Miscellaneous. Photophobia, blurred vision, increased intraocular pressure, mydriasis, anhidrosis, heat intolerance, exfoliative rash, and hypersensitivity responses including anaphylaxis

Bretylium Tosylate (Bretylol)

Pharmacology

Adrenergic blocking agent with Vaughn-Williams class III antiarrhythmic properties

Initially liberates norepinephrine from sympathetic ganglia and postganglionic adrenergic neurons—may therefore produce increased blood pressure, heart rate, cardiac output, and ventricular irritability via shortening of action potential, effective refractory period, and conduction times

Subsequent mechanism of action is to impair neuronal release and reuptake of norepinephrine by producing adrenergic blockade—this commonly produces vasodilation with hypotension, also raises threshold for ventricular fibrillation, and may decrease substrate for ventricular reentrant rhythms by increasing action potential duration and effective refractory period

May have direct vasodilator, cardiostimulant, and weak anesthetic effects

Increases sensitivity to circulating and infused catecholamines

Administrative Guidelines

Administer infusion via precision control device

Monitor ECG and blood pressure continuously

Closely follow serum electrolytes, calcium, magnesium, and acid-base status

Always dilute before use and infuse over at least 8 minutes (except bolus administration in ventricular fibrillation)—may cause nausea and vomiting if infused too rapidly

Patients should remain supine until tolerance to hypotensive effects is noted. Thereafter, observe for postural hypotension. Employ norepinephrine or dopamine and volume replacement if systolic pressure is <75 mmHg

Decrease dose in patients with renal failure

Intramuscular administration of 5 mL undiluted drug per site is acceptable if no IV line is present during therapy for ventricular fibrillation

(continued below)

Indications

Short-term prophylaxis and treatment of ventricular fibrillation

Life-threatening ventricular dysrhythmias unresponsive to first- and second-line therapy according to ACLS guidelines

Unlabeled Uses. Ventricular tachydysrhythmias associated with digitalis glycoside toxicity or quinidine use

(continued on page 38)

Contraindicated in patients with known hypersensitivity and as monotherapy in severely hypotensive patients

Use cautiously in patients on digitalis or those with severe pulmonary hypertension or significant aortic stenosis

Overdosage may manifest initially with hypertension followed by protracted hypotension. Employ nitroprusside for elevated pressure and volume plus vasodepressors such as norepinephrine for hypotension. Bretylium is removed by hemodialysis, but this may be ineffective in treating overdosage

Bretylium Tosylate (Bretylol)

Pharmacokinetics

Onset of Action. Several minutes for ventricular fibrillation; 20 minutes–2 hours for other ventricular dysrhythmias

Peak Effects. Variable, probably 6–9 hours

Duration of Action. 20 min–2 hours after IV bolus; 6–24 hours for IV infusion

IV Bolus (Distribution) Half-Life. Approximately 30 min

IV Infusion (Elimination) Half-Life. 4–17 hours. With severe renal failure 32–105 hours

Metabolism. Drug is not metabolized but excreted unchanged in urine

Dosing Information

Initial Loading Dose (Ventricular Fibrillation). 5 mg/kg ***undiluted*** IV bolus over 1 minute—may repeat 5–10 mg/kg bolus at 5–30 minute intervals for persistent ventricular fibrillation. Maximum dose is 30–35 mg/kg

Initial Loading Dose (Ventricular Tachyardia). 5–10 mg/kg ***diluted*** in 50 mL 5% dextrose in water USP over 8–10 minutes. May repeat every 1–2 hours as necessary if dysrhythmia persists

Maintenance Infusion Regimen. 1–2 mg/min continuous infusion or 5–10 mg/kg ***diluted*** over 10 minutes by intermittent infusion at 6-hour intervals

Maximum Infusion Rate. 2 mg/min

Maximum Dose. 40 mg/kg/day total dose

Titration Guideline

Suggested Regimen. Adjust infusion by 1 mg/min as required for dysrhythmia control

(continued on page 40)

Potential Drug Interactions

Possibly Potentiated by Bretylium. Digitalis, catecholamines; variable effects may be noted when used in conjunction with other antiarrhythmic drugs

Principal Adverse Effects

CNS. Vertigo, dizziness, light-headedness, syncope

CV. Postural hypotension, hypotension, increased ventricular dysrhythmias, bradycardia, angina, transient hypertension

GI. Nausea, vomiting, diarrhea, especially after rapid IV bolus

Miscellaneous. Nasal congestion

Bretylium Tosylate (Bretylol)

How Supplied

IV Injection

50 mg/mL—10-mL ampuls, vials, and syringes of 500 mg, and 20-mL vials of 1000 mg

Premixed IV Infusion

2 mg/mL—500 mg in 250-mL 5% dextrose injection USP

4 mg/mL—1 g (250 mL) or 2 g (500 mL) 5% dextrose injection USP

Bretylium Tosylate (Bretylol) 2 g in 500 mL

■ **Infusion Rate in mL/hr (pump setting)** ■ **Drug Dose in mg/min**

mL/hr	mg/min	mL/hr	mg/min	mL/hr	mg/min	mL/hr	mg/min	mL/hr	mg/min	mL/hr	mg/min
1	0.07	21	1.40	41	2.73	61	4.07	81	5.40	101	6.73
2	0.13	22	1.47	42	2.80	62	4.13	82	5.47	102	6.80
3	0.20	23	1.53	43	2.87	63	4.20	83	5.53	103	6.87
4	0.27	24	1.60	44	2.93	64	4.27	84	5.60	104	6.93
5	0.33	25	1.67	45	3.00	65	4.33	85	5.67	105	7.00
6	0.40	26	1.73	46	3.07	66	4.40	86	5.73	106	7.07
7	0.47	27	1.80	47	3.13	67	4.47	87	5.80	107	7.13
8	0.53	28	1.87	48	3.20	68	4.53	88	5.87	108	7.20
9	0.60	29	1.93	49	3.27	69	4.60	89	5.93	109	7.27
10	0.67	30	2.00	50	3.33	70	4.67	90	6.00	110	7.33
11	0.73	31	2.07	51	3.40	71	4.73	91	6.07	111	7.40
12	0.80	32	2.13	52	3.47	72	4.80	92	6.13	112	7.47
13	0.87	33	2.20	53	3.53	73	4.87	93	6.20	113	7.53
14	0.93	34	2.27	54	3.60	74	4.93	94	6.27	114	7.60
15	1.00	35	2.33	55	3.67	75	5.00	95	6.33	115	7.67
16	1.07	36	2.40	56	3.73	76	5.07	96	6.40	116	7.73
17	1.13	37	2.47	57	3.80	77	5.13	97	6.47	117	7.80
18	1.20	38	2.53	58	3.87	78	5.20	98	6.53	118	7.87
19	1.27	39	2.60	59	3.93	79	5.27	99	6.60	119	7.93
20	1.33	40	2.67	60	4.00	80	5.33	100	6.67	120	8.00

Bretylium Tosylate (Bretylol) 4 g in 500 mL

■ Infusion Rate in mL/hr (pump setting) ■ Drug Dose in mg/min

mL/hr	mg/min	mL/hr	mg/min	mL/hr	mg/min	mL/hr	mg/min	mL/hr	mg/min	mL/hr	mg/min
1	0.13	21	2.80	41	5.47	61	8.13	81	10.80	101	13.47
2	0.27	22	2.93	42	5.60	62	8.27	82	10.93	102	13.60
3	0.40	23	3.07	43	5.73	63	8.40	83	11.07	103	13.73
4	0.53	24	3.20	44	5.87	64	8.53	84	11.20	104	13.87
5	0.67	25	3.33	45	6.00	65	8.67	85	11.33	105	14.00
6	0.80	26	3.47	46	6.13	66	8.80	86	11.47	106	14.13
7	0.93	27	3.60	47	6.27	67	8.93	87	11.60	107	14.27
8	1.07	28	3.73	48	6.40	68	9.07	88	11.73	108	14.40
9	1.20	29	3.87	49	6.53	69	9.20	89	11.87	109	14.53
10	1.33	30	4.00	50	6.67	70	9.33	90	12.00	110	14.67
11	1.47	31	4.13	51	6.80	71	9.47	91	12.13	111	14.80
12	1.60	32	4.27	52	6.93	72	9.60	92	12.27	112	14.93
13	1.73	33	4.40	53	7.07	73	9.73	93	12.40	113	15.07
14	1.87	34	4.53	54	7.20	74	9.87	94	12.53	114	15.20
15	2.00	35	4.67	55	7.33	75	10.00	95	12.67	115	15.33
16	2.13	36	4.80	56	7.47	76	10.13	96	12.80	116	15.47
17	2.27	37	4.93	57	7.60	77	10.27	97	12.93	117	15.60
18	2.40	38	5.07	58	7.73	78	10.40	98	13.07	118	15.73
19	2.53	39	5.20	59	7.87	79	10.53	99	13.20	119	15.87
20	2.67	40	5.33	60	8.00	80	10.67	100	13.33	120	16.00

Calcium Chloride

Pharmacology

Hypertonic solution that provides elemental calcium required to maintain essential physiological processes

Promotes hemostasis, regulates cell membrane and capillary permeability, aids in uptake and binding of amino acids; governs release and storage of hormones and neurotransmitters, facilitates contraction of muscle and nerve impulse transmission, regulates cyanocobalamin (B_{12}) absorption and gastrin secretion, preserves the integrity of the skeletal system

Highest source of ionized calcium (273 mg or 13.6 mEq) on a per gram basis compared to calcium gluconate (93 mg or 4.65 mEq) and calcium gluceptate (90 mg or 4.5 mEq)

Administrative Guidelines

Continuously monitor ECG and vital signs

Carefully follow serum electrolytes, calcium, magnesium, and acid-base status—do not allow serum calcium levels to exceed 12 mg/dL

Administer via central line, if possible, or small needle inserted into large vein

Intracardiac injection is not routinely recommended

Never administer subcutaneously or intramuscularly

Do not admix with carbonates, sulfates, phosphates, tartrates, and tetracycline

Warm solution to body temperature if time permits

Maintain patient in a supine position

Immediately discontinue infusion if extravasation or perivascular infiltration occurs—inject 1% procaine hydrochloride into affected area and consider application of heat and coadministration of 150 units of hyaluronidase into involved site

(continued below)

Indications

Management of severe hypocalcemia, hypermagnesemia, or hyperkalemia

Prophylaxis against hypocalcemia during transfusion with citrated blood or in patients with intestinal malabsorption syndrome

Adjunctive therapy for lead poisoning, gastrointestinal or renal colic, abdominal cramps secondary to arthropod stings, and reduction of capillary permeability in allergic and hypersensitivity reactions

During advanced cardiac life support ***only*** when toxicity from hyperkalemia, hypocalcemia, or calcium channel blocker overdose is life-threatening. Routine use for enhancing myocardial contractility or coarsening ventricular fibrillation is ***not*** recommended

Unlabeled Uses. Antagonism of neuromuscular blockade from aminoglycosides, diagnosis of Zollinger-Ellison syndrome and medullary carcinoma of the thyroid, counteraction of hypotension and toxicity of calcium channel blockers

(continued on page 46)

May produce transient elevations of 11-hydroxycorticosteroids and false-negative urinary and serum magnesium values

Contraindicated with hypercalcemia, suspected or proven digitalis toxicity, and ventricular fibrillation

Use with caution in sarcoidosis, renal or cardiac disease, digitalized patients, conditions associated with hypercalcemia, acidosis, cor pulmonale, or respiratory failure

Overdosage may manifest as weakness, lethargy, refractory nausea and vomiting, coma, and death. Manage with supportive measures, sodium chloride infusion, and furosemide to promote renal clearance of calcium

Calcium Chloride

Pharmacokinetics

Onset of Action. Almost immediately

Peak Effects. 2–10 minutes

Duration of Action. 30 minutes–2 hours

Metabolism. Unabsorbed calcium is excreted mainly in feces with remainder eliminated in the urine. Absorbed calcium enters extracellular fluid and then skeletal tissue

Dosing Information*

During ACLS. Initial dose of 2–4 mg/kg intravenously over 2 minutes or 2.7 mEq (2 mL of 10% solution). Average cumulative dose range: 7–14 mEq (5–10 mL of 10% solution). Repeat initial dose every 10 minutes as necessary

Hyperkalemia. 2.7–14 mEq (2–10 mL of 10% solution) IV—may repeat in 1–2 minutes if indicated

Hypermagnesemia. 7 mEq (5 mL of 10% solution) slow IV push—subsequent doses may be required based on patient response

Hypocalcemic Tetany. 4.5–16 mEq (3–12 mL of 10% solution) IV until a therapeutic response is observed

Citrated Blood Transfusion. 1.36 mEq (1 mL of 10% solution) for each 100 mL of blood transfused

***The manufacturer recommends *not exceeding* 1 mL/min IV bolus**

(continued on page 48)

Potential Drug Interactions

Potentiation of Calcium Effects. Thiazides, digitalis glycosides

Possibly Potentiated by Calcium. Digitalis preparations

Possibly Antagonized by Calcium. Tetracycline, atenolol, verapamil, and sodium polystyrene sulfonate

Principal Adverse Effects

CV. Hypotension, dysrhythmias including bradycardia, syncope, cardiac arrest

Dermatological. Phlebitis, cellulitis, skin sloughing and necrosis at injection site, burning

Miscellaneous. Metallic taste, heat sensation, tingling

Calcium Infusion Test for Zollinger-Ellison Syndrome. 0.25 mEq/kg/hr for 3 hours. Determine serum gastrin 30 minutes before, at initiation of, and 30 minutes after infusion. A 50% rise or 500 pg/mL is abnormal

Calcium Infusion for Medullary Thyroid Carcinoma. Administer 7 mEq (5 mL of 10% solution) IV over 5–10 minutes and measure plasma calcitonin concentrations

Normal Plasma Calcium

8.5–10.5 mg/dL

How Supplied

10% (1.36 mEq/mL)—10-mL ampuls, vials, and syringes of 13.6 mEq (1 g)

Diazepam (Valium)

Pharmacology

Benzodiazepine, which exerts CNS effects at the hypothalamic, limbic, and thalamic levels—possibly via neurotransmitter inhibition of gamma-aminobutyric acid

Diminishes anxiety and promotes sedation, hypnosis, amnesia, and skeletal muscle relaxation; acts as an anticonvulsant by reducing seizure spread rather than abolishing the focus; decreases REM sleep

No significant primary effects on the peripheral autonomic, respiratory, or cardiovascular systems

Indications

Management of anxiety states

Skeletal muscle relaxation in spastic disorders

Prophylaxis in acute alcohol withdrawal syndromes

Anticonvulsant therapy in patients with status epilepticus and severe recurrent seizure disorders

Induction of sedation, light anesthesia, and amnesia before endoscopic procedures, cardioversion, or surgery

Administrative Guidelines

Administer infusion via precision control device

Administer via central line, if possible, or large vein. Do not use small veins of the hand or wrist as severe thrombophlebitis may occur

Never infuse by arterial routes as gangrene may ensue

Do not mix or dilute diazepam with other medications or infusion fluids. When direct IV injection is not feasible, inject slowly via infusion tubing as close as possible to vein insertion site

Carefully monitor vital signs during use and ensure that emergency resuscitative equipment is immediately available

When given concomitantly with narcotics, the narcotic dosage should be reduced by at least one-third

Diazepam is not intended for use as primary maintenance therapy of seizures or depressive disorders

(continued below)

Pharmacokinetics

Onset of Action. 15 minutes after IV bolus

Peak Effects. Usually within 15 minutes

Duration of Action. 15 minutes–1 hour

Metabolism. Via liver and excretion by the kidneys

Physical dependence is possible and a withdrawal syndrome may occur in cases of long-term use

Observe patients for at least 3 hours following intravenous administration and caution against operating hazardous machinery or motor vehicles, or activities requiring complete mental alertness

Contraindicated in narrow-angle or untreated open-angle glaucoma, known hypersensitivity, psychoses, shock, coma, and alcohol intoxication with depressed vital signs

Use with caution in elderly or debilitated patients; those with decreased pulmonary reserve; impaired hepatic or renal function, during obstetrical delivery; in patients given narcotics, barbiturates, or alcohol; and in individuals performing hazardous occupational work or mental acuity tasks

Overdosage typically manifests as diminished reflexes, somnolence, confusion, and coma. Manage with general supportive measures, gastric lavage followed by activated charcoal, and vasopressors for severe hypotension. Dialysis is of limited value

Diazepam (Valium)

Dosing Information

Moderate Anxiety. 2–5 mg IV—may repeat in 3–4 hours as necessary

Severe Anxiety. 5–10 mg IV—may repeat in 3–4 hours as necessary

Muscle Spasm. 5–10 mg IV—may repeat in 3–4 hours as necessary. Tetanus may require higher doses

Acute Alcohol Withdrawal. 10 mg IV initially—may repeat in 3–4 hours as necessary

Status Epilepticus. 5–10 mg IV—may repeat in 10–15 minutes as necessary up to 30 mg total dose

Cardioversion. 5–15 mg IV within 5–10 minutes before procedure

Endoscopy. 5–10 mg IV before procedure—may repeat to a total dose of 20 mg. Titrate to desired sedative response

Do not administer faster than 5 mg/min or exceed 30 mg over any 8-hour period

(continued below)

Potential Drug Interactions

Potentiation of Diazepam Effects. Disulfiram, cimetidine, alcohol, oral contraceptives, valproic acid, narcotics, phenothiazines, monoamine oxidase inhibitors, antihistamines, tricyclic antidepressants, barbiturates, psychotropics, isoniazid, anticonvulsants, CNS depressants

Antagonism of Diazepam Effects. Rifampin

Possibly Potentiated by Diazepam. Digoxin

Possibly Antagonized by Diazepam. Levodopa

Lower total doses (2–5 mg) are recommended for elderly and debilitated patients and when other sedative drugs are used

How Supplied

5 mg/mL—1-mL vials, syringes, and cartridge needle units of 5 mg

Principal Adverse Effects

CNS. Altered states of consciousness, hallucinations, ataxia, drowsiness, fatigue, headache, depression, dysarthria, tremor, vertigo, syncope, vivid dreams, paradoxical CNS stimulation including muscle spasticity, insomnia, rage, anxiety, hyperexcitable states, nystagmus, diplopia, tonic status epilepticus

Pulmonary. Dyspnea, respiratory depression, laryngospasm, apnea, cough, hyperventilation

CV. Bradycardia, hypotension, tachycardia, chest pain

GI. Nausea, constipation, dry mouth, anorexia

GU. Incontinence, urinary retention, altered libido

Allergic. Urticaria, rash, pruritus, photosensitivity, nonthrombocytopenic purpura

Miscellaneous. Phlebitis and thrombosis at injection site, hiccoughs, fever, paresthesias, gynecomastia, joint pain, leukopenia, and blood dyscrasias

Diazepam (Valium) 50 mg in 500 mL

■ **Infusion Rate in mL/hr (pump setting)** ■ **Drug Dose in mg/hr**

mL/hr	mg/hr	mL/hr	mg/hr	mL/hr	mg/hr	mL/hr	mg/hr	mL/hr	mg/hr	mL/hr	mg/hr
1	0.10	21	2.10	41	4.10	61	6.10	81	8.10	101	10.10
2	0.20	22	2.20	42	4.20	62	6.20	82	8.20	102	10.20
3	0.30	23	2.30	43	4.30	63	6.30	83	8.30	103	10.30
4	0.40	24	2.40	44	4.40	64	6.40	84	8.40	104	10.40
5	0.50	25	2.50	45	4.50	65	6.50	85	8.50	105	10.50
6	0.60	26	2.60	46	4.60	66	6.60	86	8.60	106	10.60
7	0.70	27	2.70	47	4.70	67	6.70	87	8.70	107	10.70
8	0.80	28	2.80	48	4.80	68	6.80	88	8.80	108	10.80
9	0.90	29	2.90	49	4.90	69	6.90	89	8.90	109	10.90
10	1.00	30	3.00	50	5.00	70	7.00	90	9.00	110	11.00
11	1.10	31	3.10	51	5.10	71	7.10	91	9.10	111	11.10
12	1.20	32	3.20	52	5.20	72	7.20	92	9.20	112	11.20
13	1.30	33	3.30	53	5.30	73	7.30	93	9.30	113	11.30
14	1.40	34	3.40	54	5.40	74	7.40	94	9.40	114	11.40
15	1.50	35	3.50	55	5.50	75	7.50	95	9.50	115	11.50
16	1.60	36	3.60	56	5.60	76	7.60	96	9.60	116	11.60
17	1.70	37	3.70	57	5.70	77	7.70	97	9.70	117	11.70
18	1.80	38	3.80	58	5.80	78	7.80	98	9.80	118	11.80
19	1.90	39	3.90	59	5.90	79	7.90	99	9.90	119	11.90
20	2.00	40	4.00	60	6.00	80	8.00	100	10.00	120	12.00

Infusion Rate in mL/hr (pump setting)	Drug Dose in mg/hr	Infusion Rate in mL/hr (pump setting)	Drug Dose in mg/hr	Infusion Rate in mL/hr (pump setting)	Drug Dose in mg/hr	Infusion Rate in mL/hr (pump setting)	Drug Dose in mg/hr	Infusion Rate in mL/hr (pump setting)	Drug Dose in mg/hr	Infusion Rate in mL/hr (pump setting)	Drug Dose in mg/hr
1	0.20	21	4.20	41	8.20	61	12.20	81	16.20	101	20.20
2	0.40	22	4.40	42	8.40	62	12.40	82	16.40	102	20.40
3	0.60	23	4.60	43	8.60	63	12.60	83	16.60	103	20.60
4	0.80	24	4.80	44	8.80	64	12.80	84	16.80	104	20.80
5	1.00	25	5.00	45	9.00	65	13.00	85	17.00	105	21.00
6	1.20	26	5.20	46	9.20	66	13.20	86	17.30	106	21.20
7	1.40	27	5.40	47	9.40	67	13.40	87	17.40	107	21.40
8	1.60	28	5.60	48	9.60	68	13.60	88	17.60	108	21.60
9	1.80	29	5.80	49	9.80	69	13.80	89	17.80	109	21.80
10	2.00	30	6.00	50	10.00	70	14.00	90	18.00	110	22.00
11	2.20	31	6.20	51	10.20	71	14.20	91	18.20	111	22.20
12	2.40	32	6.40	52	10.40	72	14.40	92	18.40	112	22.40
13	2.60	33	6.60	53	10.60	73	14.60	93	18.60	113	22.60
14	2.80	34	6.80	54	10.80	74	14.80	94	18.80	114	22.80
15	3.00	35	7.00	55	11.00	75	15.00	95	19.00	115	23.00
16	3.20	36	7.20	56	11.20	76	15.20	96	19.20	116	23.20
17	3.40	37	7.40	57	11.40	77	15.40	97	19.40	117	23.40
18	3.60	38	7.60	58	11.60	78	15.60	98	19.60	118	23.60
19	3.80	39	7.80	59	11.80	79	15.80	99	19.80	119	23.80
20	4.00	40	8.00	60	12.00	80	16.00	100	20.00	120	24.00

Digoxin (Lanoxin)

Pharmacology

Cardiac glycoside with direct dose-related myocardial effects and indirect actions mediated by the autonomic nervous system—vagomimetic, sympatholytic, and carotid sinus responses

Augments force and velocity of cardiac contractions (positive inotropic effect), slows heart rate (negative chronotropic effect), and decreases atrioventricular node conduction (negative dromotropic effect)

In patients with congestive heart failure, enhances cardiac output and lowers left ventricular, end diastolic, pulmonary, and systemic venous pressures—usually no adverse effects on coronary blood flow or myocardial oxygen consumption

Inhibits sodium potassium–activated ATPase

Increases CNS sympathetic stimulation of cardiac and peripheral sympathetic nerves in higher doses

Administrative Guidelines

Carefully monitor ECG and vital signs—follow serum electrolytes, calcium, and renal chemistries during use

Correct serum potassium, magnesium, and calcium, if possible, before therapy (potassium and magnesium deficiency and hypercalcemia sensitize the myocardium to digoxin)

Avoid parenteral use unless oral dosing is not feasible or urgent digitalization is essential

Decrease dose in renal failure—reduce or discontinue dose if toxic symptoms or signs are observed

Adverse effects and toxicity do not always correlate with serum drug levels. Toxicity is unlikely at levels below 0.8 ng/mL and relatively common at levels above 2.0 ng/mL

Serum levels should be measured at least 6–10 hours after the last dose and immediately before the next dose

(continued below)

Indications

Management of congestive heart failure primarily due to left ventricular systolic dysfunction

Control of ventricular rate in atrial tachydysrhythmias—atrial fibrillation, flutter, and paroxysmal atrioventricular node reentrant tachycardia (may convert the last to normal sinus rhythm)

Pharmacokinetics

Onset of Action. 5–30 minutes after IV bolus

Peak Effects. 1–5 hours

Duration of Action. 3–4 days

Plasma (Distribution) Half-Life. Approximately 30 minutes

Tissue (Elimination) Half-Life. 34–44 hours with normal renal function; 4–5 days or longer in anephric patients

Metabolism. 50–70% of dose is excreted unchanged in urine based on glomerular filtration rate

Patients with atrial fibrillation and flutter may require and tolerate higher doses than other patients

Contraindicated with known hypersensitivity, ventricular fibrillation, advanced sinoatrial or atrioventricular node block without a functioning artificial ventricular pacemaker, beriberi, some cases of carotid sinus hypersensitivity, for treatment of obesity, or treatment of sinus tachycardia in the absence of heart failure

Use with caution in acute carditis, acute glomerulonephritis, renal dysfunction, acute myocardial infarction, myxedema, hypokalemia, idiopathic hypertrophic subaortic stenosis, amyloid heart disease, Wolff-Parkinson-White and sick sinus syndromes, before electrical cardioversion, in constrictive pericarditis, Stokes-Adams attacks, severe obstructive pulmonary disease and cor pulmonale, suspected digitalis toxicity, obesity, severe heart failure, hypertension, ventricular dysrhythmias, hypocalcemia, hypomagnesemia, and atrial dysrhythmias associated with hyperthyroidism and other hypermetabolic states

(continued on page 58)

Overdosage requires continuous monitoring; supportive measures; and correction of cation deficiencies, acid-base status, and fluid balance. Discontinue digoxin and aggravating agents such as catecholamines. Consider digoxin antibody fragments for life-threatening dysrhythmias unresponsive to conventional therapeutic measures. There is no established role for dialysis in overdosage cases

Dosing Information

Initial Dose. 0.25–0.5 mg IV bolus over 5 minutes

Loading Dose Range. 1.0–1.5 mg total

Daily Maintenance Dose. 25–35% total loading dose

Administer bolus doses over at least 5 minutes to avoid systemic and coronary arterial vasoconstriction

Loading Dose Guidelines

Administer 0.125–0.25 mg IV bolus doses every 2–8 hours as necessary

$$\text{Daily maintenance dose} = \text{loading dose} \times \frac{\text{\% daily loss}}{100}$$

$$\text{Where \% daily loss} = 14 + \frac{\text{creatinine clearance}}{5}$$

Therapeutic Serum Level

0.5–2.0 ng/mL

Potential Drug Interactions

Potentiation of Digoxin Effects. Hypercalcemia, IV calcium, quinidine, calcium channel blockers, corticosteroids, diuretics, beta-blockers, succinylcholine, amiodarone, procainamide, disopyramide, lidocaine, sympathomimetics, flecainide, rauwolfia alkaloids, insulin, propantheline, hydroxychloroquine, alpha-adrenergic blockers, diphenoxylate

Antagonism of Digoxin Effects. Hypocalcemia, penicillamine, thyroid hormone, magnesium and potassium salts (except in advanced heart block), antigen-binding Fab fragments, antacids, kaolin-pectin, neomycin, cholestyramine, sulfasalazine, and some anticancer drugs

Digoxin (Lanoxin)

How Supplied

0.25 mg/mL—1-mL Tubex of 0.25 mg
2-ml ampuls, vials, and Tubex of 0.50 mg

Principal Adverse Effects

CNS. Headache, visual disturbances (yellow or blurred vision), weakness, apathy, psychosis, depression, altered mental status, seizures, aphasia, hallucinations, paresthesias, facial pain, disturbing dreams

CV. Extrasystoles, ventricular tachydysrhythmias, junctional rhythms, heart block, sinus node dysfunction, paroxysmal atrial tachycardia with varying block

GI. Nausea, vomiting, diarrhea, anorexia, abdominal pain, intestinal necrosis

Allergic. Rash, thrombocytopenia, eosinophilia

Miscellaneous. Gynecomastia, muscle weakness, hyperkalemia

Digoxin Immune Fab (Digibind)

Pharmacology

Antigen binding fragments that bind to free digoxin or digitoxin in both intravascular and extracellular fluid

Competitively blocks and reverses the inhibition of NA^+ and K^+-ATPase activity produced by digoxin and digitoxin

Electrophysiologic toxic effects of digitalis preparations are more rapidly reversed than inotropic toxic effects

Affinity greater for digoxin than digitoxin. Efficacy for other digoxin derivatives uncertain

Administrative Guidelines

Administer infusion via precision control device

Add 4 mL sterile water for injection to each vial yielding a concentration of 10 mg/mL. Then infuse within 4 hours through a 0.22-μm membrane filter

Monitor the ECG continuously and carefully follow vital signs

Obtain serum digoxin/digitoxin levels before use—values obtained within 6–10 hours of oral ingestion are probably inaccurate

Carefully follow the serum K^+ concentrations before and after Digibind administration

Determine allergic history before use of Digibind. Protein allergy or previous treatment with Digibind may increase risk of hypersensitivity reactions

Consider skin or scratch testing before use in high-risk individuals for allergy. Employ 10 μg/mL reconstituted dose intradermally and observe at 20 minutes for urticarial wheal and erythema

(continued below)

Indications

Adjunctive therapy in the management of life-threatening digoxin or digitoxin intoxication

Severe cardiac glycoside toxicity associated with serum K^+ levels of 5.0 mEq/L or greater

Severe cardiac glycoside toxicity in the setting of at least 10 mg digoxin ingestion

Unlabeled Uses. Antidote for all digitalis glycoside preparations; prophylaxis against life-threatening episodes of glycoside intoxication; and diagnosis of cardiac glycoside toxicity

Consider toxicity from other drugs in suicidal ingestion or if no response is noted

Avoid potassium supplementation or catecholamine use if possible

Each 40-mg vial binds 0.6 mg of digoxin or digitoxin

Total serum digoxin levels frequently rise 10-fold to 20-fold following Digibind use but are not clinically reliable. Elevated levels are secondary to biologically inactive Fab-digoxin complexes

Accurate serum glycoside levels require clearance of Fab fragments by the kidney (usually 2–7 days)

Do not redigitalize for 2–7 days, if possible, until Digibind is completely eliminated

Monitor functionally anephric patients for a prolonged period of time for recurrent cardiac glycoside toxicity

Serum potassium levels generally return to normal values within 2–6 hours. Beware of possible hypokalemia secondary to intracellular potassium shifts

Cardiac dysrhythmias are usually controlled within 3 hours

(continued on page 64)

Digoxin Immune Fab (Digibind)

Pharmacokinetics

Onset of Action. Usually within 30 minutes. Varies according to infusion rate, dose administered, and amount of glycoside to be bound

Peak Effects. Within 30 minutes

Duration of Action. Approximately 8–12 hours

Elimination Half-Life. 14–20 hours with normal renal function

Metabolism. Renal elimination by glomerular filtration

Extracardiac effects, such as drowsiness, nausea, and vomiting, also resolve within 3–6 hours

No known ***contraindications***

Use with caution in patients with renal impairment, known hypersensitivity, and poor cardiac function (may exacerbate heart failure)

Overdosage effects have not been fully elucidated. Observe for allergic responses, fever, or delayed serum sickness reaction

Dosing Information

Infusion Rate. Determine appropriate dose and administer over 15–30 minutes

Imminent Cardiac Arrest. Determine appropriate dose and administer by rapid IV bolus injection

1. Glycoside level is known: see Table A
2. Glycoside level is unknown but patient on oral therapy: 240 mg (6 vials)
3. Amount of glycoside ingested known: see Table B
4. Amount of glycoside ingested unknown: 800 mg (20 vials)

May repeat dose in several hours if toxicity is not reversed

How Supplied

Single-use vials of **40 mg**

Potential Drug Interactions

Possibly Antagonized by Digibind. Digoxin, digitoxin, and possibly other cardiac glycosides

Possibly Potentiated by Digibind. Warfarin

Principal Adverse Effects

CV. Heart failure, rapid ventricular response in patients with atrial fibrillation

Dermatological. Urticarial rash, erythema at infusion site

Allergic. Anaphylaxis

Miscellaneous. Hypokalemia

TABLE A Adult Dose Estimate of Digibind (in No. of Vials) from Serum Digoxin Concentration

		Serum Digoxin Concentration (ng/mL)						
		1	**2**	**4**	**8**	**12**	**16**	**20**
Patient Weight (kg)	**40**	0.5v	1v	2v	3v	5v	6v	8v
	60	0.5v	1v	2v	5v	7v	9v	11v
	70	1v	2v	3v	5v	8v	11v	13v
	80	1v	2v	3v	6v	9v	12v	15v
	100	1v	2v	4v	8v	11v	15v	19v

Reproduced with permission of Burroughs Wellcome Co., Research Triangle Park, NC
v = vials

TABLE B Approximate Digibind Dose for Reversal of a Single Ingestion Digoxin Overdose

Number of Digoxin Tablets or Capsules Ingested*	Digibind Dose	
	mg	No. of Vials
25	340	8.5
50	680	17
75	1000	25
100	1360	34
150	2000	50
200	2680	67

*0.25 mg tablets with 80% bioavailability or 0.2 mg Lanoxicaps Capsules
Reproduced with permission of Burroughs Wellcome Co., Research Triangle Park, NC

Diltiazem Hydrochloride (Cardizem)

Pharmacology

Inhibits calcium ion influx across membranes of cardiac and vascular smooth muscle cells

Slows atrioventricular nodal conduction and prolongs atrioventricular nodal refractoriness, thereby slowing ventricular response in atrial fibrillation and flutter

May slow sinus node discharge rate, especially in those with disturbed sinus node function

Decreases systolic and diastolic blood pressure by decreasing total peripheral resistance

May decrease myocardial contractility, especially in patients with impaired ventricular function

May decrease coronary vascular tone and antagonize coronary spasm

Administrative Guidelines

Administer infusion via precision control device

Carefully monitor ECG and vital signs

Incompatible when mixed directly with furosemide solution

Consider initiation of oral antiarrhythmic therapy within 3 hours of IV dosing

Contraindicated in atrial fibrillation or flutter associated with an accessory bypass tract, within a few hours of IV beta-blocker use, those with ventricular tachycardia, severe hypotension or shock, sick sinus syndrome in the absence of a functioning artificial ventricular pacemaker, second-degree or third-degree block unless a functioning artificial ventricular pacemaker is present, acute myocardial infarction, and those with known hypersensitivity

Use cautiously in patients with hepatic or renal dysfunction, the elderly, those with heart failure or compromised ventricular function, patients taking drugs

(continued below)

Indications

Control of heart rate in atrial fibrillation and flutter with rapid ventricular response in the absence of an accessory bypass tract

Conversion of paroxysmal supraventricular tachycardia to sinus rhythm, even in the presence of an accessory bypass tract

Pharmacokinetics

Onset of Action. Within 3 minutes

Peak Effects. 2–7 minutes

Duration of Action. 1–3 hours after single IV bolus, 0.5–10 hours after cessation of infusion

Elimination Half-Life. 3.4 hours after IV bolus

Metabolism. Almost completely by liver with excretion in urine and bile primarily as inactive metabolites

that decrease peripheral resistance, myocardial contractility, sinoatrial or atrioventricular conduction disturbances, intravascular volume depletion, and hypotension

Overdosage should be managed with appropriate supportive measures, including atropine or isuprel, pacing for high-grade block and bradycardia, vasopressors for hypotension, and inotropes and diuretics for heart failure

Diltiazem Hydrochloride (Cardizem)

Dosing Information

Initial IV Bolus Dose. 0.25 mg/kg over 2 minutes

Repeat Bolus Dosing. If initial clinical response inadequate, administer second bolus of 0.35 mg/kg over 2 minutes. Additional IV bolus dosing may be required on an individual basis

Initial Infusion Rate. 5–10 mg/hour

Maintenance Infusion Range. 5–15 mg/hour

Maximal Infusion Rate. 15 mg/hour

Titration Guideline

Suggested Regimen. Adjust infusion by 5 mg/hour as required to control heart rate

How Supplied

5 mg/mL—5-mL vials of 25 mg

10 mg/mL—10-mL vials of 50 mg

Potential Drug Interactions

Potentiation of Diltiazem Effects. Digitalis preparations, H_2 receptor blockers, beta-blockers, ionic contrast media, anesthetics, drugs that depress sinoatrial or atrioventricular node conduction, drugs metabolized by the cytochrome P-450 oxidase pathway.

Antagonism of Diltiazem Effects. Calcium

Possibly Potentiated by Diltiazem. Anesthetics, digitalis, beta-blockers

Principal Adverse Effects

CNS. Paresthesias, dizziness
CV. Hypotension, junctional rhythm or isorhythmic atrioventricular dissociation, heart block, sinus node dysfunction, chest pain, heart failure, syncope, ventricular dysrhythmias, atrial flutter
GI. Nausea, vomiting, constipation, and elevated liver enzymes
Dermatological. Flushing, injection site reaction, pruritus
Miscellaneous. Diaphoresis, headache, dyspnea, edema, amblyopia, dry mouth, asthenia, hyperuricemia

Diltiazem Hydrochloride (Cardizem) 125 mg in 500 mL

■ Infusion Rate in mL/hr (pump setting) ■ Drug Dose in mg/hr

mL/hr	mg/hr	mL/hr	mg/hr	mL/hr	mg/hr	mL/hr	mg/hr	mL/hr	mg/hr	mL/hr	mg/hr
1	0.25	21	5.25	41	10.25	61	15.25	81	20.25	101	25.25
2	0.50	22	5.50	42	10.50	62	15.50	82	20.50	102	25.50
3	0.75	23	5.75	43	10.75	63	15.75	83	20.75	103	25.75
4	1.00	24	6.00	44	11.00	64	16.00	84	21.00	104	26.00
5	1.25	25	6.25	45	11.25	65	16.25	85	21.25	105	26.25
6	1.50	26	6.50	46	11.50	66	16.50	86	21.50	106	26.50
7	1.75	27	6.75	47	11.75	67	16.75	87	21.75	107	26.75
8	2.00	28	7.00	48	12.00	68	17.00	88	22.00	108	27.00
9	2.25	29	7.25	49	12.25	69	17.25	89	22.25	109	27.25
10	2.50	30	7.50	50	12.50	70	17.50	90	22.50	110	27.50
11	2.75	31	7.75	51	12.75	71	17.75	91	22.75	111	27.75
12	3.00	32	8.00	52	13.00	72	18.00	92	23.00	112	28.00
13	3.25	33	8.25	53	13.25	73	18.25	93	23.25	113	28.25
14	3.50	34	8.50	54	13.50	74	18.50	94	23.50	114	28.50
15	3.75	35	8.75	55	13.75	75	18.75	95	23.75	115	28.75
16	4.00	36	9.00	56	14.00	76	19.00	96	24.00	116	29.00
17	4.25	37	9.25	57	14.25	77	19.25	97	24.25	117	29.25
18	4.50	38	9.50	58	14.50	78	19.50	98	24.50	118	29.50
19	4.75	39	9.75	59	14.75	79	19.75	99	24.75	119	29.75
20	5.00	40	10.00	60	15.00	80	20.00	100	25.00	120	30.00

Diltiazem Hydrochloride (Cardizem) 250 mg in 250 mL

■ Infusion Rate in mL/hr (pump setting) ■ Drug Dose in mg/hr

mL/hr	mg/hr	mL/hr	mg/hr	mL/hr	mg/hr	mL/hr	mg/hr	mL/hr	mg/hr	mL/hr	mg/hr
1	1.0	21	21.0	41	41.0	61	61.0	81	81.0	101	101.0
2	2.0	22	22.0	42	42.0	62	62.0	82	82.0	102	102.0
3	3.0	23	23.0	43	43.0	63	63.0	83	83.0	103	103.0
4	4.0	24	24.0	44	44.0	64	64.0	84	84.0	104	104.0
5	5.0	25	25.0	45	45.0	65	65.0	85	85.0	105	105.0
6	6.0	26	26.0	46	46.0	66	66.0	86	86.0	106	106.0
7	7.0	27	27.0	47	47.0	67	67.0	87	87.0	107	107.0
8	8.0	28	28.0	48	48.0	68	68.0	88	88.0	108	108.0
9	9.0	29	29.0	49	49.0	69	69.0	89	89.0	109	109.0
10	10.0	30	30.0	50	50.0	70	70.0	90	90.0	110	110.0
11	11.0	31	31.0	51	51.0	71	71.0	91	91.0	111	111.0
12	12.0	32	32.0	52	52.0	72	72.0	92	92.0	112	112.0
13	13.0	33	33.0	53	53.0	73	73.0	93	93.0	113	113.0
14	14.0	34	34.0	54	54.0	74	74.0	94	94.0	114	114.0
15	15.0	35	35.0	55	55.0	75	75.0	95	95.0	115	115.0
16	16.0	36	36.0	56	56.0	76	76.0	96	96.0	116	116.0
17	17.0	37	37.0	57	57.0	77	77.0	97	97.0	117	117.0
18	18.0	38	38.0	58	58.0	78	78.0	98	98.0	118	118.0
19	19.0	39	39.0	59	59.0	79	79.0	99	99.0	119	119.0
20	20.0	40	40.0	60	60.0	80	80.0	100	100.0	120	120.0

Dobutamine Hydrochloride (Dobutrex)

Pharmacology

Synthetic derivative of dopamine that does not release endogenous norepinephrine

Primary effect is inotropic stimulation of the heart principally by $beta_1$-adrenergic mechanism and possibly $alpha_1$-adrenergic activity

Increases cardiac output, coronary blood flow, and myocardial oxygen consumption. May decrease pulmonary vascular resistance

Mild vasodilator ($beta_2$) effects, which can reduce peripheral resistance and cause hypotension

Minimal vasoconstrictor ($alpha_1$) stimulation usually seen at high doses

Facilitates atrioventricular conduction and has mild chronotropic and arrhythmogenic properties

Administrative Guidelines

Carefully monitor blood pressure, ECG, and, if possible, hemodynamic variables. Consider potassium monitoring because hypokalemia may occur

Infusion solution may display some pink discoloration (owing to drug oxidation), which does not require discarding or discontinuation

Do not admix with other drugs, especially bicarbonate, heparin, some cephalosporins, penicillin, and other alkaline solutions

Correct any underlying hypovolemia, if possible, before use

Patients in atrial fibrillation should be digitalized before use (may accelerate ventricular response)

Decrease or discontinue infusion if excessive hypotension, hypertension, tachycardia, or dysrhythmias ensue

Synergistic improvement in cardiac output may occur with nitroprusside, dopamine, or phosphodiesterase inhibitors such as amrinone

(continued below)

Indications

Short-term inotropic management of patients with depressed cardiac contractility, including those with right ventricular infarction

Unlabeled Use. During acute myocardial infarction

Pharmacokinetics

Onset of Action. 1–2 minutes

Peak Effects. 1–10 minutes

Duration of Action. Less than 10 minutes

Mean Plasma Half-Life. 2 minutes

Metabolism. Principally via liver to an inactive compound, which is excreted in urine and feces

Contraindicated as monotherapy in severely hypovolemic patients, idiopathic hypertrophic subaortic stenosis, and known hypersensitivity

Use cautiously in patients with hypertension, ventricular ectopy, or acute myocardial infarction (may intensify ischemia via increased cardiac work)

Overdosage usually manifests as excessive change in blood pressure or tachycardia. Manage by reducing infusion rate or temporarily discontinuing the drug, and provide general supportive measures

Dobutamine Hydrochloride (Dobutrex)

Dosing Information

Initial Infusion Rate. 2.5 μg/kg/min

Maintenance Infusion Range. 2.5–10 μg/kg/min

Maximal Infusion Rate. 40 μg/kg/min

Titration Guideline

Suggested Regimen. Adjust infusion by 2.5 μg/kg/min every 10 minutes as required

How Supplied

12.5 mg/mL—20-mL vials (250 mg)

Potential Drug Interactions

Potentiation of Dobutamine Effects. Nitroprusside, cyclopropane, halogenated hydrocarbon anesthetics, oxytocic agents, monoamine oxidase inhibitors, tricyclic antidepressants, guanethidine, bretylium

Antagonism of Dobutamine Effects. Beta-blockers

Possibly Antagonized by Dobutamine. Insulin

Principal Adverse Effects

CNS. Headache, paresthesias

CV. Excessive increases in heart rate, blood pressure, or ventricular ectopy; dose-related chest pain and shortness of breath

GI. Nausea, vomiting

Dermatological. Phlebitis

Miscellaneous. Leg cramps, pruritus of scalp

Dobutamine Hydrochloride (Dobutrex) 500 mg in 500 mL

DRUG DOSE in µg/kg/min

Infusion Rate in mL/hr \ Patient's Weight kg/lbs	40/88	45/99	50/110	55/121	60/132	65/143	70/154	75/165	80/176	85/187	90/198	95/209	100/220	105/231	110/242
5	2.1	1.9	1.7	1.5	1.4	1.3	1.2	1.1	1.0	1.0	0.9	0.9	0.8	0.8	0.8
10	4.2	3.7	3.3	3.0	2.8	2.6	2.4	2.2	2.1	2.0	1.9	1.8	1.7	1.6	1.5
15	6.2	5.6	5.0	4.5	4.2	3.8	3.6	3.3	3.1	2.9	2.8	2.6	2.5	2.4	2.3
20	8.3	7.4	6.7	6.1	5.6	5.1	4.8	4.4	4.2	3.9	3.7	3.5	3.3	3.2	3.0
25	10.4	9.3	8.3	7.6	6.9	6.4	6.0	5.6	5.2	4.9	4.6	4.4	4.2	4.0	3.8
30	12.5	11.1	10.0	9.1	8.3	7.7	7.1	6.7	6.2	5.9	5.6	5.3	5.0	4.8	4.5
35	14.6	13.0	11.7	10.6	9.7	9.0	8.3	7.8	7.3	6.9	6.5	6.1	5.8	5.6	5.3
40	16.7	14.8	13.3	12.1	11.1	10.3	9.5	8.9	8.3	7.8	7.4	7.0	6.7	6.3	6.1
45	18.7	16.7	15.0	13.6	12.5	11.5	10.7	10.0	9.4	8.8	8.3	7.9	7.5	7.1	6.8
50	20.8	18.5	16.7	15.2	13.9	12.8	11.9	11.1	10.4	9.8	9.3	8.8	8.3	7.9	7.6
55	22.9	20.4	18.3	16.7	15.3	14.1	13.1	12.2	11.5	10.8	10.2	9.6	9.2	8.7	8.3
60	25.0	22.2	20.0	18.2	16.7	15.4	14.3	13.3	12.5	11.8	11.1	10.5	10.0	9.5	9.1
65	27.1	24.1	21.7	19.7	18.1	16.7	15.5	14.4	13.5	12.7	12.0	11.4	10.8	10.3	9.3
70	29.2	25.9	23.3	21.2	19.4	17.9	16.7	15.6	14.8	13.7	13.0	12.3	11.7	11.1	10.6
75	31.2	27.8	25.0	22.7	20.8	19.2	17.9	16.7	15.6	14.7	13.9	13.2	12.5	11.9	11.4
80	33.3	29.6	26.7	24.2	22.2	20.5	19.0	17.8	16.7	15.7	14.8	14.0	13.3	12.7	12.1
85	35.4	31.5	28.3	25.8	23.6	21.8	20.2	18.9	17.7	16.7	15.7	14.9	14.2	13.5	12.9
90	37.5	33.3	30.0	27.3	25.0	23.1	21.4	20.0	18.7	17.6	16.7	15.8	15.0	14.3	13.6
95	39.6	35.2	31.7	28.8	26.4	24.4	22.6	21.1	19.8	18.6	17.6	16.7	15.8	15.1	14.4
100	41.7	37.0	33.3	30.3	27.8	25.6	23.8	22.2	20.8	19.6	18.5	17.5	16.7	15.9	15.2
105	43.7	38.9	35.0	31.8	29.2	26.9	25.0	23.3	21.9	20.6	19.4	18.4	17.5	16.7	15.9
110	45.8	40.7	36.7	33.3	30.6	28.2	26.2	24.4	22.9	21.6	20.4	19.3	18.3	17.5	16.7
115	47.9	42.6	38.3	34.8	31.9	29.5	27.4	25.6	24.0	22.5	21.3	20.2	19.2	18.3	17.4
120	50.0	44.4	40.0	36.4	33.3	30.8	28.6	26.7	25.0	23.5	22.2	21.1	20.0	19.0	18.2

DRUG DOSE in µg/kg/min

Patient's Weight kg	40	45	50	55	60	65	70	75	80	85	90	95	100	105	110
lbs	88	99	110	121	132	143	154	165	176	187	198	209	220	231	242
Infusion Rate in mL/hr															
5	4.2	3.7	3.3	3.0	2.8	2.6	2.4	2.2	2.1	2.0	1.9	1.8	1.7	1.6	1.5
10	8.3	7.4	6.7	6.1	5.6	5.1	4.8	4.4	4.2	3.9	3.7	3.5	3.3	3.2	3.0
15	12.5	11.1	10.0	9.1	8.3	7.7	7.1	6.7	6.3	5.9	5.6	5.3	5.0	4.8	4.5
20	16.7	14.8	13.3	12.1	11.1	10.3	9.5	8.9	8.3	7.8	7.4	7.0	6.7	6.3	6.1
25	20.8	18.5	16.7	15.2	13.9	12.8	11.9	11.1	10.4	9.8	9.3	8.8	8.3	7.9	7.6
30	25.0	22.2	20.0	18.2	16.7	15.4	14.3	13.3	12.5	11.8	11.1	10.5	10.0	9.5	9.1
35	29.2	25.9	23.3	21.2	19.4	17.9	16.7	15.6	14.6	13.7	13.0	12.3	11.7	11.1	10.6
40	33.3	29.6	26.7	24.2	22.2	20.5	19.0	17.8	16.7	15.7	14.8	14.0	13.3	12.7	12.1
45	37.5	33.3	30.0	27.3	25.0	23.1	21.4	20.0	18.8	17.6	16.7	15.8	15.0	14.3	13.6
50	41.7	37.0	33.3	30.3	27.8	25.6	23.8	22.2	20.8	19.6	18.5	17.5	16.7	15.9	15.2
55	45.8	40.7	36.7	33.3	30.6	28.2	26.2	24.4	22.9	21.6	20.4	19.3	18.3	17.5	16.7
60	50.0	44.4	40.0	36.4	33.3	30.8	28.6	26.7	25.0	23.5	22.2	21.1	20.0	19.0	18.2
65	54.2	48.1	43.3	39.4	36.1	33.3	31.0	28.9	27.1	25.5	24.1	22.8	21.7	20.6	19.7
70	58.3	51.9	46.7	42.4	38.9	35.9	33.3	31.1	29.2	27.5	25.9	24.6	23.3	22.2	21.2
75	62.5	55.6	50.0	45.5	41.7	38.5	35.7	33.3	31.3	29.4	27.8	26.3	25.0	23.8	22.7
80	66.7	59.3	53.3	48.5	44.4	41.0	38.1	35.6	33.3	31.4	29.6	28.1	26.7	25.4	24.2
85	70.8	63.0	56.7	51.5	47.2	43.6	40.5	37.8	35.4	33.3	31.5	29.8	28.3	27.0	25.8
90	75.0	66.7	60.0	54.5	50.0	46.2	42.9	40.0	37.5	35.3	33.3	31.6	30.0	28.6	27.3
95	79.2	70.4	63.3	57.6	52.8	48.7	45.2	42.2	39.6	37.3	35.2	33.3	31.7	30.2	28.8
100	83.3	74.1	66.7	60.6	55.6	51.3	47.6	44.4	41.7	39.2	37.0	35.1	33.3	31.7	30.3
105	87.5	77.8	70.0	63.6	58.3	53.8	50.0	46.7	43.8	41.2	38.9	36.8	35.0	33.3	31.8
110	91.7	81.5	73.3	66.7	61.1	56.4	52.4	48.9	45.8	43.1	40.7	38.6	36.7	34.9	33.3
115	95.8	85.2	76.7	69.7	63.9	59.0	54.8	51.1	47.9	45.1	42.6	40.4	38.3	36.5	34.8
120	100.0	88.9	80.0	72.7	66.7	61.5	57.1	53.3	50.0	47.1	44.4	42.1	40.0	38.1	36.4

Dopamine Hydrochloride (Intropin)

Pharmacology

Endogenous catecholamine precursor of norepinephrine that stimulates adrenergic receptors of the sympathetic nervous system

Alpha-adrenergic and beta-adrenergic effects are mediated by inhibition and activation of adenyl cyclase (influences cyclic AMP production)

Releases norepinephrine from storage sites

Dilates renal, mesenteric, coronary, and intracerebral vascular beds by activation of dopaminergic receptors at low doses (<2 μg/kg/min). May increase renal blood flow, glomerular filtration rate, sodium excretion, and urine output

Moderate doses (2–10 μg/kg/min) stimulate beta$_1$-receptors to increase heart rate, cardiac output, coronary blood flow, and myocardial oxygen consumption. Blood pressure and pulmonary vascular effects are variable

May facilitate atrioventricular conduction and excitability and induce dysrhythmias

(continued below)

Administrative Guidelines

Administer infusion via precision control device

Carefully monitor blood pressure, ECG, hemodynamics, renal function, and acid-base status

Carefully observe infusion site for free-flow, blanching, and extravasation

Administer via central line, if possible, or large vein

Do not admix with alkaline solutions, bicarbonates, oxidizing drugs, or iron salts

Always dilute before use

Correct any underlying hypovolemia, acidosis, hypercapnia, and hypoxia before or concurrently with use

Decrease or discontinue infusion in the presence of declining renal function, vasoconstriction, significant dysrhythmias, or excessive rise in blood pressure

Suggest concomitant norepinephrine use if doses greater than 20 μg/kg/min required for blood pressure

(continued below)

Alpha$_1$ effects predominate at higher doses (>10 µg/kg/min) and may result in renal and mesenteric vasoconstriction and an elevated peripheral vascular resistance

No significant effect on beta$_2$-adrenergic receptors

Indications

Augmentation of cardiac performance, blood pressure, and renal blood flow in early shock and hypoperfusion syndromes owing to septicemia, refractory cardiac failure, cardiac surgery, trauma, and acute myocardial infarction

Unlabeled Uses. Hepatorenal syndrome, acute renal failure; cirrhosis; and barbiturate, meprobamate, or salicylate intoxication

Consider phentolamine mesylate 5–10 mg IV to prevent renal vasoconstriction with higher doses

When discontinuing infusion in patients receiving >5 µg/kg/min, the final dosage should not be less than 5 µg/kg/min to avoid recurrent hypotension. Prepare to infuse IV fluids if necessary

Extravasation requires discontinuation of drug and immediate subcutaneous infiltraton of 5–10 mg phentolamine in 10–15 mL saline

Contraindicated in patients with pheochromocytoma, uncorrected tachyarrhythmias, ventricular fibrillation, or known hypersensitivity and ***as sole therapy in hypovolemic patients***

Use cautiously in patients with ischemic heart disease and peripheral vascular disease. Decrease or discontinue infusion if limb ischemia observed. Consider 5–10 mg IV phentolamine mesylate and, although unproven, 10 mg of chlorpromazine IV followed by 0.6 mg/min chlorpromazine infusion

(continued on page 82)

Dopamine Hydrochloride (Intropin)

Pharmacokinetics

Onset of Action. 2–5 minutes

Peak Effects. 2–10 minutes

Duration of Action. Less than 10 minutes

Plasma (Distribution) Half-Life. Approximately 2 minutes

Metabolism. Via liver, kidneys, and plasma, including approximately 25% metabolized to norepinephrine. Excreted by the kidneys

Overdosage typically produces excessive blood pressure elevation. Decrease or discontinue infusion, and consider short-acting alpha-blockade with phentolamine mesylate

Dosing Information

Initial Infusion Rate. 1–5 μg/kg/min

Severe Vascular Occlusive Disease. 0.5–1 μg/kg/min

Severely Ill Patients. 5 μg/kg/min

Maintenance Infusion Range. Up to 20 μg/kg/min

Maximum Infusion Rate. Rarely greater than 50 μg/kg/min

Titration Guideline

Suggested Regimen. Adjust infusion by 1–4 μg/kg/min every 10–30 minutes as required; increments of 5–10 μg/kg/min may be necessary in severely ill patients

Potential Drug Interactions

Potentiation of Dopamine Effects. Monoamine oxidase inhibitors, tricyclic antidepressants, diuretics, cyclopropane or halogenated hydrocarbon anesthetics, oxytocic agents

Antagonism of Dopamine Effects. Beta-blockers and alpha-blockers

Possibly Antagonized by Dopamine. Guanethidine, phenytoin, and dopamine may lead to bradycardia, hypotension, and seizures

Dopamine Hydrochloride (Intropin)

How Supplied

IV Injection

40 mg/mL—5-mL ampuls, vials, and syringes of 200 mg
10-mL vials and syringes of 400 mg
20-mL vials of 800 mg

80 mg/mL—5-mL ampuls, vials, and syringes of 400 mg
10-mL syringes of 800 mg
20-mL vials of 1600 mg

160 mg/mL—5-mL ampuls, vials, and syringes of 800 mg

Premixed IV Infusion

0.8 mg/mL—250 mL (200 mg) and 500 mL (400 mg) 5% dextrose injection USP

1.6 mg/mL—250 mL (400 mg) and 500 mL (800 mg) 5% dextrose injection USP

3.2 mg/mL—250 mL (800 mg) and 500 mL (1600 mg) 5% dextrose injection USP

Principal Adverse Effects

CNS. Headache, dilated pupils, anxiety

CV. Hypotension, vasoconstriction, ectopic beats and tachydysrhythmias, chest pain, limb ischemia, hypertension, brachycardia, widened QRS, dyspnea, palpitations, conduction abnormalities

GI. Nausea, vomiting

Renal. Azotemia

Dermatological. Skin sloughing and necrosis at infusion site

Miscellaneous. Elevation of serum glucose

Dopamine Hydrochloride (Intropin) 400 mg in 500 mL

DRUG DOSE in µg/kg/min

Patient's Weight kg / lbs	40 / 88	45 / 99	50 / 110	55 / 121	60 / 132	65 / 143	70 / 154	75 / 165	80 / 176	85 / 187	90 / 198	95 / 209	100 / 220	105 / 231	110 / 242
Infusion Rate in mL/hr															
5	1.7	1.5	1.3	1.2	1.1	1.0	1.0	0.9	0.8	0.8	0.7	0.7	0.7	0.6	0.6
10	3.3	3.0	2.7	2.4	2.2	2.1	1.9	1.8	1.7	1.6	1.5	1.4	1.3	1.3	1.2
15	5.0	4.4	4.0	3.6	3.3	3.1	2.9	2.7	2.5	2.4	2.2	2.1	2.0	1.9	1.8
20	6.7	5.9	5.3	4.8	4.4	4.1	3.8	3.6	3.3	3.1	3.0	2.8	2.7	2.5	2.4
25	8.3	7.4	6.7	6.1	5.6	5.1	4.8	4.4	4.2	3.9	3.7	3.5	3.3	3.2	3.0
30	10.0	8.9	8.0	7.3	6.7	6.2	5.7	5.3	5.0	4.7	4.4	4.2	4.0	3.8	3.6
35	11.7	10.4	9.3	8.5	7.8	7.2	6.7	6.2	5.8	5.5	5.2	4.9	4.7	4.4	4.2
40	13.3	11.9	10.7	9.7	8.9	8.2	7.6	7.1	6.7	6.3	5.9	5.6	5.3	5.1	4.8
45	15.0	13.3	12.0	10.9	10.0	9.2	8.6	8.0	7.5	7.1	6.7	6.3	6.0	5.7	5.5
50	16.7	14.8	13.3	12.1	11.1	10.3	9.5	8.9	8.3	7.8	7.4	7.0	6.7	6.3	6.1
55	18.3	16.3	14.7	13.3	12.2	11.3	10.5	9.8	9.2	8.6	8.1	7.7	7.3	7.0	6.7
60	20.0	17.8	16.0	14.5	13.3	12.3	11.4	10.7	10.0	9.4	8.9	8.4	8.0	7.6	7.3
65	21.7	19.3	17.3	15.8	14.4	13.3	12.4	11.6	10.8	10.2	9.6	9.1	8.7	8.3	7.9
70	23.3	20.7	18.7	17.0	15.6	14.4	13.3	12.4	11.7	11.0	10.4	9.8	9.3	8.9	8.5
75	25.0	22.2	20.0	18.2	16.7	15.4	14.3	13.3	12.5	11.8	11.1	10.5	10.0	9.5	9.1
80	26.7	23.7	21.3	19.4	17.8	16.4	15.2	14.2	13.3	12.5	11.9	11.2	10.7	10.2	9.7
85	28.3	25.2	22.7	20.6	18.9	17.4	16.2	15.1	14.2	13.3	12.6	11.9	11.3	10.8	10.3
90	30.0	26.7	24.0	21.8	20.0	18.5	17.1	16.0	15.0	14.1	13.3	12.6	12.0	11.4	10.9
95	31.7	28.1	25.3	23.0	21.1	19.5	18.1	16.9	15.8	14.9	14.1	13.3	12.7	12.1	11.5
100	33.3	29.8	26.7	24.2	22.2	20.5	19.0	17.8	16.7	15.7	14.8	14.0	13.3	12.7	12.1
105	35.0	31.1	28.0	25.5	23.3	21.5	20.0	18.7	17.5	16.5	15.6	14.7	14.0	13.3	12.7
110	36.7	32.6	29.3	26.7	24.4	22.6	21.0	19.6	18.3	17.3	16.3	15.4	14.7	14.0	13.3
115	38.3	34.1	30.7	27.9	25.6	23.6	21.9	20.4	19.2	18.0	17.0	16.1	15.3	14.6	13.9
120	40.0	35.6	32.0	29.1	26.7	24.6	22.9	21.3	20.0	18.8	17.8	16.8	16.0	15.2	14.5

DRUG DOSE in μg/kg/min

Infusion Rate in ml/hr	Patient's Weight kg / lbs: 40 / 88	45 / 99	50 / 110	55 / 121	60 / 132	65 / 143	70 / 154	75 / 165	80 / 176	85 / 187	90 / 198	95 / 209	100 / 220	105 / 231	110 / 242
5	3.3	3.0	2.7	2.4	2.2	2.1	1.9	1.8	1.7	1.6	1.5	1.4	1.3	1.3	1.2
10	6.7	5.9	5.3	4.8	4.4	4.1	3.8	3.6	3.3	3.1	3.0	2.8	2.7	2.5	2.4
15	10.0	8.9	8.0	7.3	6.7	6.2	5.7	5.3	5.0	4.7	4.4	4.2	4.0	3.8	3.6
20	13.3	11.9	10.7	9.7	8.9	8.2	7.6	7.1	6.7	6.3	5.9	5.6	5.3	5.1	4.8
25	16.7	14.8	13.3	12.1	11.1	10.3	9.5	8.9	8.3	7.8	7.4	7.0.	6.7	6.3	6.1
30	20.0	17.8	16.0	14.5	13.3	12.3	11.4	10.7	10.0	9.4	8.9	8.4	8.0	7.6	7.3
35	23.3	20.7	18.7	17.0	15.6	14.4	13.3	12.4	11.7	11.0	10.4	9.8	9.3	8.9	8.5
40	26.7	23.7	21.3	19.4	17.8	16.4	15.2	14.2	13.3	12.5	11.9	11.2	10.7	10.2	9.7
45	30.0	26.7	24.0	21.8	20.0	18.5	17.1	16.0	15.0	14.1	13.3	12.6	12.0	11.4	10.9
50	33.3	29.6	26.7	24.2	22.2	20.5	19.0	17.8	16.7	15.7	14.8	14.0	13.3	12.7	12.1
55	36.7	32.6	29.3	26.7	24.4	22.6	21.0	19.6	18.3	17.3	16.3	15.4	14.7	14.0	13.3
60	40.0	35.6	32.0	29.1	26.7	24.6	22.9	21.3	20.0	18.8	17.8	16.8	16.0	15.2	14.5
65	43.3	38.5	34.7	31.5	28.9	26.7	24.8	23.1	21.7	20.4	19.3	18.2	17.3	16.5	15.8
70	46.7	41.5	37.3	33.9	31.1	28.7	26.7	24.9	23.3	22.0	20.7	19.6	18.7	17.8	17.0
75	50.0	44.4	40.0	36.4	33.3	30.8	28.6	26.7	25.0	23.5	22.2	21.1	20.0	19.0	18.2
80	53.3	47.4	42.7	38.8	35.6	32.8	30.5	28.4	26.7	25.1	23.7	22.5	21.3	20.3	19.4
85	56.7	50.4	45.3	41.2	37.8	34.9	32.4	30.2	28.3	26.7	25.2	23.9	22.7	21.6	20.6
90	60.0	53.3	48.0	43.6	40.0	36.9	34.3	32.0	30.0	28.2	26.7	25.3	24.0	22.9	21.8
95	63.3	56.3	50.7	46.1	42.2	39.0	36.2	33.8	31.7	29.8	28.1	26.7	25.3	24.1	23.0
100	66.7	59.3	53.3	48.5	44.4	41.0	38.1	35.6	33.3	31.4	29.6	28.1	26.7	25.4	24.2
105	70.0	62.2	56.0	50.9	46.7	43.1	40.0	37.3	35.0	32.9	31.1	29.5	28.0	26.7	25.5
110	73.3	65.2	58.7	53.3	48.9	45.1	41.9	39.1	36.7	34.5	32.6	30.9	29.3	27.9	26.7
115	76.7	68.1	61.3	55.8	51.1	47.2	43.8	40.9	38.3	36.1	34.1	32.3	30.7	29.2	27.9
120	80.0	71.1	64.0	58.2	53.3	49.2	45.7	42.7	40.0	37.6	35.6	33.7	32.0	30.5	29.1

Enalaprilat

Pharmacology

Prevents conversion of angiotensin I to angiotensin II by inhibiting angiotensin converting enzyme (ACE)

Decreases blood pressure by reduced peripheral vascular resistance

May decrease aldosterone levels, increase plasma renin activity, inhibit norepinephrine release, and increase circulating bradykinin

May cause venodilation and reduce pulmonary artery and pulmonary capillary wedge pressures

May increase renal blood flow, glomerular filtration rate, BUN, creatinine, and serum potassium

No significant effects on heart rate, stroke volume, or cardiac output—rarely produces orthostasis

Administrative Guidelines

Carefully follow electrolytes, renal function, and vital signs in patients with hypovolemia, with sodium depletion, those on diuretics or dialysis, and with heart failure

Decrease IV bolus dose by 50% to 0.625 mg in patients with severe renal impairment or those on dialysis

Begin oral therapy at 5 mg daily for those on 1.25 mg enalaprilat every 6 hours

Discontinue immediately if angioedema occurs

Contraindicated in those with known hypersensitivity or history of angioedema secondary to ACE therapy

Use with caution in those with renal dysfunction, especially with known or suspected renovascular hypertension, in patients with hypovolemia, with sodium depletion, those on diuretics or dialysis, and with heart failure

(continued below)

Indications

Management of mild to severe hypertension when oral therapy is not practical. Treatment of heart failure unresponsive to digitalis preparation and diuretics

Unlabeled Uses. Prevention of left ventricular dilatation following acute infarction and control of hypertensive crisis

Pharmacokinetics

Onset of Action. 5–15 minutes

Peak Effects. 1–4 hours

Duration of Action. Approximately 6 hours

Elimination Half-Life. 30–87 hours

Metabolism. About 90% excreted as unchanged drug in urine

Overdosage may manifest as severe hypotension, stupor, renal failure, hyponatremia, and hyperkalemia. Manage with supportive measures and consider dialysis if necessary

Enalapril at

Drug Information

Initial Dose. 1.25 mg IV over 5 minutes in patients not receiving a diuretic. 0.625 mg IV over 5 minutes in patients receiving diuretics. May repeat after 1 hour if inadequate response

Subsequent IV Dosing. 1.25 mg IV every 6 hours

Maximum IV Bolus Dose. Up to 5 mg every 6 hours

Maximum Daily Dose. 20 mg

How Supplied

1.25 mg/mL—1-mL vial of 1.25 mg
2-mL vial of 2.5 mg

Potential Drug Interactions

Potentiation of Enalaprilat Effects. Diuretics and agents promoting renin release, potassium, and potassium sparing drugs

Possibly Potentiated by Enalaprilat. Lithium

Principal Adverse Effects

CNS. Headache, dizziness, altered mental status, neuropathy, nervousness

Pulmonary. Dyspnea, bronchospasm, cough, pneumonia, bronchitis

CV. Hypotension, hypertension, myocardial infarction, angina, dysrhythmias, pulmonary embolism, pulmonary edema, cardiac arrest, chest pain

GI. Nausea, constipation, ileus, pancreatitis, hepatic dysfunction, bleeding, vomiting, dyspepsia, anorexia

Heme. Neutropenia, thrombocytopenia, marrow depression, hemolysis

(continued below)

Allergic. Angioedema, anaphylaxis, fever, lupuslike syndrome, rash

Renal. Oliguria, renal failure

Dermatological. Exfoliative dermatitis, Stevens-Johnson syndrome, erythema multiforme, pruritus, alopecia, photosensitivity

Miscellaneous. Increased BUN and creatinine, hypokalemia and hyperkalemia, elevated liver enzymes, minor decreases in hemoglobin and hematocrit

Epinephrine 1:1000 (Adrenalin)

Pharmacology

Endogenous catecholamine produced by the adrenal medulla, which stimulates both alpha-adrenergic and beta-adrenergic receptors

Alpha-adrenergic and beta-adrenergic effects are mediated by inhibition and activation of adenyl cyclase (influences cyclic AMP production)

Beta effects predominate with small-to-moderate doses—relaxes bronchial smooth muscle (beta$_2$ effect), gastrointestinal smooth muscle, and smooth muscle of the iris. Produces positive chronotropic and inotropic (beta$_1$) cardiac response, which increases cardiac output, heart rate, blood pressure (mainly systolic), and coronary blood flow. Dilates skeletal muscle vasculature and may increase cerebral blood flow owing to elevated blood pressure

Alpha effects noted with higher doses, including constriction of bronchial arteries and renal arteries, reduced blood flow to skin, mucosa, and splanchnic

(continued below)

Administrative Guidelines

Administer infusion via precision control device

Continuously monitor vital signs, ECG, hemodynamic variables, renal function, and acid-base status

Carefully observe infusion site for free-flow, blanching, and extravasation

Administer via central line, if possible, or large vein

Protect from light and discard if pinkish or brown color noted or precipitate observed

Endotracheal tube and intracardiac administration should be reserved only in extreme emergencies when IV access is not in place

Correct underlying hypovolemia, if possible, before use

Beta-adrenergic receptor effects persist after alpha-adrenergic effects dissipate and may produce hypotension

Tolerance may develop with prolonged use

(continued below)

circulation; and elevation of peripheral vascular resistance and blood pressure

Reduces bronchospasm, pulmonary congestion, and edema; increases vital capacity and tidal volume

Inhibits histamine release and end organ effects; increases lipolysis and serum free fatty acid, cholesterol, and lipid levels; augments serum glucose by blocking insulin release and glucose reuptake by liver and enhancing glycogenolysis

May increase serum potassium, lactate levels, and oxygen consumption, and inhibits uterine contractions, especially during the second stage of labor

Rarely produces apnea by direct respiratory center inhibition

Extravasation requires discontinuation of drug and immediate subcutaneous infiltration of 5–10 mg phentolamine in 10–15 mL saline

Contraindicated in setting of known hypersensitivity, narrow-angle glaucoma, nonanaphylactic shock, cerebral arteriosclerosis or organic brain damage, labor, local anesthesia to distal extremities, general anesthesia with chloroform, trichloroethylene, cyclopropane or halogenated hydrocarbons, acute coronary insufficiency, organic heart disease or cardiac dilatation, digitalis toxicity, and phenothiazine-induced hypotension

Use cautiously in those with sensitivity to sympathomimetic agents, the elderly, Parkinson's disease, those with cardiovascular or renal disease, hypertension, diabetes mellitus, emphysema, hyperthyroidism, ventricular fibrillation, hypovolemia, or psychoneurotic disorders

Overdosage may manifest as hypertensive crisis, with apnea or pulmonary edema, and cardiac dysrhythmias. Provide general supportive measures and consider alpha-blockers or nitroprusside for excessive pressor effects

Epinephrine 1:1000 (Adrenalin)

Indications

Ventricular fibrillation and pulseless ventricular tachycardia, asystole, pulseless electrical activity (electromechanical dissociation), severe bradycardia, complete heart block, Stokes-Adams episodes, refractory asthma attacks, coarsening of ventricular fibrillation, and acute severe hypersensitivity reactions, including anaphylaxis

Unlabeled Uses. Celiac artery infusion for GI bleeding, renal artery injection to enhance visualization of contralateral kidney or to protect the kidney from radiation nephritis

Pharmacokinetics

Onset of Action. Immediate

Peak Effects. Within 3 minutes

Duration of Action. Not specified by manufacturer

IV Bolus (Distribution) Half-Life. 3 minutes

Metabolism. Via liver, sympathetic nerve endings, and other tissues to inactive metabolites, which are excreted in the urine

Dosing Information

IV Bolus Dose During Resuscitation. 1 mg (10 mL) of 1:10,000 solution every 3–5 minutes as required. Follow each peripheral dose with 20-mL flush

IV Infusion Dose During Cardiac Arrest. 100 mL/hour of 30 mg 1:1000 solution added to 250 mL of normal saline or 5% dextrose in water—titrate to desired hemodynamic end point

IV Dose for Anaphylactic Shock. 0.1–0.25 mg (1–2.5 mL) of 1:10,000 solution slow IV injection over 5–10 minutes. Repeat every 5–15 minutes as necessary or begin continuous infusion at 1 μg/min

Intracardiac Dose. 0.1–1.0 mg (1–10 mL) of 1:10,000 solution

Endotracheal Dose. 2–2.5 mg of 1:10,000 solution diluted with 10 mL of normal saline

Initial Infusion Rate for Other Situations. 1 μg/min

Maintenance Infusion Range. 1–10 μg/min

Maximum Infusion Rate. Not specified by manufacturer

Potential Drug Interactions

Potentiation of Epinephrine Effects. Sympathomimetics, tricyclic antidepressants, digitalis glycosides, antihistamines, oxytocic agents, cyclopropane, halogenated hydrocarbon anesthetics, bretylium, guanethidine

Antagonism of Epinephrine Effects. Alkalis, oxidizing agents such as nitrates, beta-blockers, alpha-blockers, phenothiazines

Epinephrine 1:1000 (Adrenalin)

Titration Guideline

Suggested Regimen. Individual responses are highly variable—adjust infusion by 1 μg/min every 5 minutes as required to achieve desired hemodynamic effects

How Supplied

1:1000 (1 mg/mL)—1-mL ampuls, vials, and syringes of 1 mg
2-mL syringes of 2 mg
30-mL vials of 30 mg

1:10,000 (0.1 mg/mL)—3-mL syringes of 0.3 mg
10-mL syringes of 1.0 mg

Principal Adverse Effects

CNS. Cerebral hemorrhage, hemiplegia, anxiety, excitability, headache, tremor, weakness, dizziness, pallor, sweating, apprehension, lightheadedness, altered consciousness, insomnia, psychosis, suicidal and homicidal ideation

Pulmonary. Respiratory weakness, respiratory distress, and apnea

CV. Palpitations, dysrhythmias, hypertension, angina, aortic rupture, pulmonary edema, syncope, peripheral and visceral vasoconstriction

GI. Nausea, vomiting, elevated aspartate aminotransferase levels

Renal. Hypervolemia, reduced urine output, renal failure, metabolic acidosis

Dermatological. Skin sloughing and necrosis at infusion site

Miscellaneous. Tachyphylaxis with prolonged use, elevated glucose, lactic acidosis

Epinephrine 1:1000 (Adrenalin) 3 mg in 250 mL

■ **Infusion Rate in mL/hr (pump setting)** ■ **Drug Dose in µg/min**

mL/hr	µg/min	mL/hr	µg/min	mL/hr	µg/min	mL/hr	µg/min	mL/hr	µg/min	mL/hr	µg/min
1	0.2	21	4.2	41	8.2	61	12.2	81	16.2	101	20.2
2	0.4	22	4.4	42	8.4	62	12.4	82	16.4	102	20.4
3	0.6	23	4.6	43	8.6	63	12.6	83	16.6	103	20.6
4	0.8	24	4.8	44	8.8	64	12.8	84	16.8	104	20.8
5	1.0	25	5.0	45	9.0	65	13.0	85	17.0	105	21.0
6	1.2	26	5.2	46	9.2	66	13.2	86	17.2	106	21.2
7	1.4	27	5.4	47	9.4	67	13.4	87	17.4	107	21.4
8	1.6	28	5.6	48	9.6	68	13.6	88	17.6	108	21.6
9	1.8	29	5.8	49	9.8	69	13.8	89	17.8	109	21.8
10	2.0	30	6.0	50	10.0	70	14.0	90	18.0	110	22.0
11	2.2	31	6.2	51	10.2	71	14.2	91	18.2	111	22.2
12	2.4	32	6.4	52	10.4	72	14.4	92	18.4	112	22.4
13	2.6	33	6.6	53	10.6	73	14.6	93	18.6	113	22.6
14	2.8	34	6.8	54	10.8	74	14.8	94	18.8	114	22.8
15	3.0	35	7.0	55	11.0	75	15.0	95	19.0	115	23.0
16	3.2	36	7.2	56	11.2	76	15.2	96	19.2	116	23.2
17	3.4	37	7.4	57	11.4	77	15.4	97	19.4	117	23.4
18	3.6	38	7.6	58	11.6	78	15.6	98	19.6	118	23.6
19	3.8	39	7.8	59	11.8	79	15.8	99	19.8	119	23.8
20	4.0	40	8.0	60	12.0	80	16.0	100	20.0	120	24.0

Infusion Rate in mL/hr (pump setting)	Drug Dose in µg/min	Infusion Rate in mL/hr (pump setting)	Drug Dose in µg/min	Infusion Rate in mL/hr (pump setting)	Drug Dose in µg/min	Infusion Rate in mL/hr (pump setting)	Drug Dose in µg/min	Infusion Rate in mL/hr (pump setting)	Drug Dose in µg/min	Infusion Rate in mL/hr (pump setting)	Drug Dose in µg/min
1	0.33	21	7.00	41	13.67	61	20.33	81	27.00	101	33.67
2	0.67	22	7.33	42	14.00	62	20.67	82	27.33	102	34.00
3	1.00	23	7.67	43	14.33	63	21.00	83	27.67	103	34.33
4	1.33	24	8.00	44	14.67	64	21.33	84	28.00	104	34.67
5	1.67	25	8.33	45	15.00	65	21.67	85	28.33	105	35.00
6	2.00	26	8.67	46	15.33	66	22.00	86	28.67	106	35.33
7	2.33	27	9.00	47	15.67	67	22.33	87	29.00	107	35.67
8	2.67	28	9.33	48	16.00	68	22.67	88	29.33	108	36.00
9	3.00	29	9.67	49	16.33	69	23.00	89	29.67	109	36.33
10	3.33	30	10.00	50	16.67	70	23.33	90	30.00	110	36.67
11	3.67	31	10.33	51	17.00	71	23.67	91	30.33	111	37.00
12	4.00	32	10.67	52	17.33	72	24.00	92	30.67	112	37.33
13	4.33	33	11.00	53	17.67	73	24.33	93	31.00	113	37.67
14	4.67	34	11.33	54	18.00	74	24.67	94	31.33	114	38.00
15	5.00	35	11.67	55	18.33	75	25.00	95	31.67	115	38.33
16	5.33	36	12.00	56	18.67	76	25.33	96	32.00	116	38.67
17	5.67	37	12.33	57	19.00	77	25.67	97	32.33	117	39.00
18	6.00	38	12.67	58	19.33	78	26.00	98	32.67	118	39.33
19	6.33	39	13.00	59	19.67	79	26.33	99	33.00	119	39.67
20	6.67	40	13.33	60	20.00	80	26.67	100	33.33	120	40.00

Esmolol Hydrochloride (Brevibloc)

Pharmacology

Short-acting cardioselective ($beta_1$) adrenergic receptor blocking agent—no appreciable bronchial or vascular smooth muscle ($beta_2$) effects at usual clinical doses (<300 μg/kg/min)

With typical clinical doses, there is no significant sympathomimetic, membrane-stabilizing, or alpha-adrenergic activity

Produces negative inotropic and chronotropic activity—decreases myocardial contractility, heart rate, arterial pressure, and cardiac oxygen consumption. May increase left ventricular end diastolic and capillary wedge pressures at high doses or with preexisting depressed ejection fractions

Vaughan-Williams class II antiarrhythmic agent, which decreases atrioventricular conduction and sinus node cycle length while prolonging sinus node recovery time

Less lipophilic than labetalol or propranolol

Administrative Guidelines

Administer infusion via precision control device

Employ central line, if possible, or large vein—avoid extravasation because skin necrosis may occur

Continually monitor heart rate and carefully follow blood pressure

Avoid infusion concentrations greater than 10 mg/mL owing to increased risk of thrombophlebitis

Always dilute before use—do not admix with diazepam, furosemide, thiopental, or sodium bicarbonate

Correct any underlying hypovolemia, if possible, before use

Safety and efficacy of infusions beyond 48 hours have not been established

(continued below)

Indications

Short-term control of rapid ventricular response in atrial fibrillation and flutter

Temporary control of heart rate in noncompensatory sinus tachycardia

Unlabeled Uses. Regulation of blood pressure associated with surgery, accelerated hypertension syndromes, and aortic dissection; management of myocardial ischemia

Pharmacokinetics

Onset of Action. 1–2 minutes

Peak Effects. Approximately 5 minutes

Duration of Action. 10–20 minutes

Plasma (Distribution) Half-Life. 2 minutes

Tissue (Elimination) Half-Life. Averages 9 minutes (range 5–23 minutes)

Without loading doses, steady-state is achieved in 10–30 minutes

Metabolism. In the cytosol of erythrocytes with nonhepatic and nonrenal elimination

During transition to oral antiarrhythmic medication, decrease infusion by 50% at 30 minutes ***after*** the first dose of the oral agent. Terminate infusion, if patient is clinically stable, 1 hour after the second dose of the oral agent has been given

Contraindicated in patients with known hypersensitivity, severe congestive heart failure, cardiogenic shock, sinus bradycardia, or second-degree or third-degree atrioventricular block

Use with caution in compensated heart failure, bronchospastic lung disease, renal impairment, acute coronary syndromes, and diabetes mellitus

Overdosage typically manifests as bradycardia or hypotension. Heart block and bronchospasm may also be seen. Manage with appropriate supportive measures and consider direct antagonism of effects with isoproterenol or glucagon. There is no established role for dialysis

Esmolol Hydrochloride (Brevibloc)

Dosing Information

Initial IV Loading Dose. 500 μg/kg over 1 minute, then infusion of 50 μg/kg/min for 4 minutes

Maintenance Infusion Range. 50–200 μg/kg/min

Maximum Infusion Rate. 300 μg/kg/min. Infusion rates beyond 200 μg/kg/min are not generally recommended

Titration Guidelines

Increase infusion by 50 μg/kg/min increments every 5 minutes as necessary

Administer additional 500 μg/kg loading dose over 1 minute ***before*** each increase of infusion

As target heart rate is approached, or adverse response is noted, decrease titration intervals from 5 to 10 minutes, omit loading dose, and reduce maintenance infusion dose increment to 25 μg/kg/min or lower as required

How Supplied

10 mg/mL—10-mL vials of 100 mg

250 mg/mL—10-mL ampuls of 2500 mg

Potential Drug Interactions

Potentiation of Esmolol Effects. Reserpine, morphine, and warfarin

Antagonism of Esmolol Effects. Isoproterenol and glucagon

Possibly Potentiated by Esmolol. Digoxin and succinylcholine

Principal Adverse Effects

CNS. Dizziness, somnolence, seizure, confusion, headache, fatigue, agitation, anxiety, anorexia, paresthesias, lightheadedness, depression, flushing, irritability, diaphoresis

Pulmonary. Bronchospasm, nasal congestion, dyspnea, wheezing

CV. Symptomatic hypotension, asymptomatic hypotension, asystole, heart block, congestive failure, peripheral ischemia, bradycardia, chest pain, syncope, pulmonary edema, diaphoresis, pallor, hypertension, ventricular extrasystoles

GI. Nausea, constipation, dry mouth, vomiting, dyspepsia, abdominal pain, anorexia, xerostomia

Dermatological. Rash, edema, erythema, infusion site burning, inflammation, phlebitis, skin necrosis

Miscellaneous. Fever, rigors, urinary retention, visual disturbances, midscapular pain

Esmolol Hydrochloride (Brevibloc) 5 g in 500 mL

DRUG DOSE in µg/kg/min

Patient's Weight kg / lbs	40 / 88	45 / 99	50 / 110	55 / 121	60 / 132	65 / 143	70 / 154	75 / 165	80 / 176	85 / 187	90 / 198	95 / 209	100 / 220	105 / 231	110 / 242
Infushion Rate in mL/hr															
5	20	18	16	15	13	12	11	11	10	9	9	8	8	7	7
10	41	37	33	30	27	25	23	22	20	19	18	17	16	15	15
15	62	55	50	45	41	38	35	33	31	29	27	26	25	23	22
20	83	74	66	60	55	51	47	44	41	39	37	35	33	31	30
25	104	92	83	75	69	64	59	55	52	49	48	43	41	39	37
30	125	111	100	90	83	76	71	66	62	58	55	52	50	47	45
35	145	129	116	106	97	89	83	77	72	68	64	61	58	55	53
40	166	148	133	121	111	102	95	88	83	78	74	70	66	63	60
45	187	166	150	136	125	115	107	100	93	88	83	78	75	71	68
50	208	185	166	151	138	128	119	111	104	98	92	87	83	79	75
55	229	203	183	168	152	141	131	122	114	107	101	96	91	87	83
60	250	222	200	181	166	153	142	133	125	117	111	105	100	95	90
65	270	240	216	197	180	166	154	144	135	127	120	114	108	103	98
70	281	259	233	212	194	179	166	155	145	137	129	122	116	111	106
75	312	277	250	227	208	192	178	166	158	147	138	131	125	119	113
80	333	296	266	242	222	205	190	177	166	156	148	140	133	127	121
85	354	314	283	257	236	217	202	188	177	166	157	149	141	134	128
90	375	333	300	272	250	230	214	200	187	176	166	157	150	142	136
95	395	351	316	287	263	243	226	211	197	186	175	166	158	150	143
100	416	370	333	303	277	256	238	222	208	196	185	175	166	158	151
105	437	388	350	318	291	269	250	233	218	205	194	184	175	166	159
110	458	407	366	333	305	282	261	244	229	215	203	193	183	174	166
115	479	425	383	348	319	294	273	255	239	225	213	201	191	182	174
120	500	444	400	363	333	307	285	266	250	235	222	210	200	190	181

DRUG DOSE in µg/kg/min

Patient's Weight kg / lbs	40 / 88	45 / 99	50 / 110	55 / 121	60 / 132	65 / 143	70 / 154	75 / 165	80 / 176	85 / 187	90 / 198	95 / 209	100 / 220	105 / 231	110 / 242
Infusion Rate in mL/hr															
5	41	37	33	30	27	25	23	22	20	19	18	17	16	15	15
10	83	74	66	60	55	51	47	44	41	39	37	35	33	31	30
15	125	111	100	90	83	76	71	66	62	58	55	52	50	47	45
20	166	148	133	121	111	102	95	88	83	78	74	70	66	63	60
25	208	185	166	151	138	128	119	111	104	98	92	87	83	79	75
30	250	222	200	181	166	153	142	133	125	117	111	105	100	95	90
35	291	259	233	212	194	179	166	155	145	137	129	122	116	111	106
40	333	296	266	242	222	205	190	177	166	156	148	140	133	127	121
45	375	333	300	272	250	230	214	200	187	176	166	157	150	142	136
50	416	370	333	303	277	256	238	222	208	196	185	175	166	158	151
55	458	407	366	333	305	282	261	244	229	215	203	193	183	174	166
60	500	444	400	363	333	307	285	266	250	235	222	210	200	190	181
65	541	481	433	393	361	333	309	288	270	254	240	228	216	206	197
70	583	518	466	424	388	359	333	311	291	274	259	245	233	222	212
75	625	555	500	454	416	384	357	333	312	294	277	263	250	238	227
80	666	592	533	484	444	410	381	355	333	313	296	280	266	254	242
85	708	629	566	515	472	435	404	377	354	333	314	298	283	269	257
90	750	666	600	545	500	461	428	400	375	352	333	315	300	285	272
95	791	703	633	575	527	487	452	422	395	372	351	333	316	301	287
100	833	740	666	606	555	512	476	444	416	392	370	350	333	317	303
105	875	777	700	636	583	538	500	466	437	411	388	368	350	333	318
110	916	814	733	666	611	564	523	488	458	431	407	386	366	349	333
115	958	851	766	697	638	589	547	511	479	451	425	403	383	365	348
120	1000	888	800	727	666	615	571	533	500	470	444	421	400	381	363

Famotidine (Pepcid)

Pharmacology

Competitively inhibits histamine effects on H_2 receptor of parietal cells, thereby reducing gastric acid secretion

Indirectly reduces pepsin secretion in a dose-dependent manner

May protect the stomach against irritant effects of aspirin and nonsteroidal anti-inflammatory drugs

No significant effects on biliary secretion, gastric emptying, or lower esophageal sphincter tone

Indications

Endoscopically or radiographically documented active duodenal ulcer

Hypersecretory pathologic GI disorders such as Zollinger-Ellison syndrome and systemic mastocytosis

Short-term management of benign active gastric ulcers

Short-term symptomatic relief of esophagitis or gastroesophageal reflux

Unlabeled Uses. Control of gastric pH and stress-induced GI bleeding in critically ill patients

Administrative Guidelines

Dilute with 0.9% sodium chloride, 0.45% sodium chloride, or 5% dextrose injection USP

Contraindicated in patients with known hypersensitivity

Use with caution and decrease dose as noted and in renal failure

Overdosage has not been reported based on manufacturer's insert. Hemodialysis is ineffective in removing famotidine

Pharmacokinetics

Onset of Action. Within 30 minutes

Peak Effects. 30 minutes–3 hours

Duration of Effects. Approximately 12 hours

Elimination Half-Life. 2.5–4 hours

Metabolism. Via the liver, although 65–80% excreted in urine as unchanged drug

Renal failure prolongs effects with elimination half-life of 24 hours in anuric patients

Famotidine (Pepcid)

Dosing Information

Initial Bolus Dose. 20 mg IV in 5–10 mL compatible solution at rate no faster than 10 mg/min

Intermittent Infusion Dose. 20 mg IV in 100 mL compatible solution over 15–30 minutes

Duodenal Ulcer. 20 mg IV every 12 hours as necessary

Hypersecretory States. 20 mg IV every 6 hours as necessary

Titration Guideline

Suggested Regimen. Adjust infusion dose intervals to maintain suitable gastric pH and clinical response. Diminish dose by approximately 50% if creatinine clearance 30–50 mL/min and by 75% if clearance less than 30 mL/min

How Supplied

10 mg/mL—2-mL single dose vials of 20 mg
4-mL multidose vials of 40 mg

Potential Drug Interaction

No significant predictable interactions reported by manufacturer's insert

Principal Adverse Effects

CNS. Headache, dizziness, seizures, weakness, parasthesias, fatigue, drowsiness, altered mental status

CV. Palpitations, dysrhythmias, atrioventricular block

GI. Diarrhea, constipation, nausea, vomiting, anorexia, dry mouth, cholestatic jaundice, abnormal liver tests, eructation, flatulence, heartburn

Renal. Proteinuria, increases in BUN and creatinine

Dermatological. Pruritus, urticaria, dry skin, acne, rash

Allergic. Anaphylaxis, bronchospasm, angioedema

Miscellaneous. Fever, arthralgia, flushing, tinnitus, hypertension, musculoskeletal pain, blood dyscrasias, including leukocytosis and pancytopenia

Flumazenil (Romazicon)

Pharmacology

Selective benzodiazepine receptor antagonist

Competitively inhibits recognition site of GABA/benzodiazepine receptor complex in the central nervous system

Indications

Reversal of benzodiazepine effects in general anesthesia, conscious sedation, and suspected or proven benzodiazepine overdose

Pharmacokinetics

Onset of Action. 1–2 minutes

Peak Effects. 6–10 minutes

Duration of Action. Variable depending on dose given and plasma level of benzodiazepine

Distribution Half-Life. 7–15 minutes

Elimination Half-Life. 41–79 minutes

Metabolism. Via liver. Clearance is diminished with hepatic dysfunction or reduced hepatic blood flow

Administrative Guidelines

Monitor blood pressure, ECG, and respirations and be prepared to manage seizures

Administer via freely running large vein to avoid irritation

Monitor for resedation, respiratory depression, and hypoventilation up to 120 minutes after use in conscious sedation or general anesthesia

Query patients about alcohol, sedative, and benzodiazepine use before administration and caution against operating hazardous machinery, motor vehicles, or activities requiring complete mental alertness following use

May precipitate seizures and withdrawal syndromes in those dependent on benzodiazepines

Amnesia is not consistently reversed

Contraindicated in patients with known hypersensitivity to benzodiazepines or flumazenil, those given benzodiazepines for management of

(continued below)

life-threatening illnesses, and patients with evidence of serious tricyclic antidepressant overdose, motor dysfunction, anticholinergic signs, or cardiovascular instability

Use with caution in head injury cases; panic disorders; those with respiratory depression; liver dysfunction; alcohol, barbiturate, or cross-tolerant sedative dependence; and nursing women. Avoid use in those on neuromuscular blocking agents until effects have been reversed, those with benzodiazepine dependence, or those with abstinence syndrome. Also avoid use in ICU to diagnose benzodiazepine-induced sedation

Overdosage may produce anxiety, agitation, hypersensitivity, increased muscle tone, and seizures. Manage with supportive measures and consider anticonvulsive therapy when indicated

Flumazenil (Romazicon)

Dosing Information

Reversal of Conscious Sedation and General Anesthesia

Initial IV Dose. 0.2 mg over 15–50 seconds

Maintenance Dose. 0.2 mg IV every 60 seconds as necessary up to 0.8 mg

Maximum Dose. 1.0 mg over 5 minutes

May repeat regimen at 20-minute intervals

Total dose not to exceed 3.0 mg in any hour

Suspected Benzodiazepine Overdosage. 0.2–0.5 mg/min up to 3.0 mg total dose

Patients Tolerant to Benzodiazepines. Consider 0.1 mg/min and lower total dose to decrease confusion and agitation

How Supplied

0.1 mg/mL—5-mL multidose vials of 0.5 mg
10-mL multidose vials of 1.0 mg

Potential Drug Interactions

Potentiation of Flumazenil Effects. None known

Antagonism of Flumazenil Effects. Benzodiazepines

Principal Adverse Effects

CNS. Seizures, agitation, emotional lability, dizziness, blurred vision, paresthesias

CV. Atrial and ventricular tachydysrhythmias, bradycardia, chest pain, hypertension, cutaneous vasodilation

GI. Nausea and vomiting, hiccups

Miscellaneous. Injection site irritation, rigors, shivering, diaphoresis, abnormal hearing, death

Heparin Sodium

Pharmacology

Anionic sulfated glycosaminoglycan present in mast cells—calcium salt derived from porcine intestinal mucosa and sodium salt prepared from bovine lung or porcine intestinal mucosa

Inhibits clotting by accelerating antithrombin III's (heparin cofactor) inactivation of factor Xa and preventing conversion of prothrombin to thrombin

Heparin-antithrombin III complex inactivates factors IX, X, Xa, XI, and XII and thrombin

Impedes conversion of fibrinogen to fibrin and prevents stable fibrin clot formation by factor XIII inactivation

Prevents thrombin-induced activation of factors V and VIII

Typically prolongs activated clotting time (ACT), activated partial thromboplastin time (APTT), prothrombin time (PT), thrombin time (TT), whole blood clotting time, and plasma recalcification time

(continued below)

Administrative Guidelines

Administer infusion via precision control device

Carefully monitor vital signs and coagulation test results—recommend every-4-hour APTT during initiation of therapy targeting for 1.5–2.5 times control value in most cases—ACT may also be used, aiming for 2–3 times control value in seconds

Perform platelet count before and during therapy—follow CBC, stool guaiacs, potassium, liver function tests, and serum lipids periodically

Discontinue infusion if hemorrhage noted (virtually any body site may be involved), significant thrombocytopenia develops, or new evidence of thrombosis ("white clot syndrome") suspected

Heparin resistance and higher doses may be required in febrile or postoperative states, cancer, acute myocardial infarction, thrombosis, thrombophlebitis, infections associated with thrombosis, pulmonary embolism, and familial antithrombin III deficiency

(continued below)

No significant fibrinolytic effects, alteration of clotting factor concentrations, or prolongation of bleeding time—variable platelet effects

May enhance clearance of plasma lipids via lipoprotein lipase and raise circulating free fatty acids

Indications

Prophylaxis and treatment of venous thrombosis, pulmonary emboli, and peripheral arterial emboli; atrial fibrillation with embolization; disseminated intravascular coagulation (DIC); prevention of clotting during arterial or open heart surgery, dialysis, extracorporeal circulation, blood transfusions, and in laboratory blood specimens

Unlabeled Uses. Acute coronary syndromes, including myocardial infarction and unstable angina; anterior transmural infarction with or without mural thrombi; before cardioversion with atrial fibrillation of at least 2 days' duration; adjunctive therapy with thrombolytics and during mechanical coronary revascularization; transient ischemic attacks and stroke in evolution

Heparin may elevate hepatic transaminases, interfere with coagulation studies (especially PT) and serum thyroxine measurements, elevate serum potassium (hypoaldosterone effect), and plasma lipids

Maintain heparin infusion for several days following therapeutic International Normalized Ratio (INR) or PT during conversion to oral anticoagulant therapy

Contraindicated with known hypersensitivity, severe thrombocytopenia, inability to monitor coagulation studies and in uncontrolled bleeding disorders (except DIC)

Use with caution in women over 60 years of age, conditions associated with a bleeding diathesis, with drugs that affect platelet function, thrombolytic agents, in diabetes, renal insufficiency, severe hepatic dysfunction, and with prior history of allergy or thrombocytopenia

Overdosage typically manifests with bleeding. Provide supportive measures, fluids, and blood products as needed. Heparin effects may be antagonized by

(continued on page 116)

Heparin Sodium

Pharmacokinetics

Onset of Action. Immediate post IV bolus

Peak Effects. Almost immediately post IV bolus

Duration of Action. Approximately 4 hours

Mean Plasma Half-Life for Anticoagulant Effect. 1–2 hours

IV Bolus (Distribution) Half-Life. 10 minutes

IV Infusion (Elimination) Half-Life. 30–180 minutes (dose dependent)

Metabolism. Via reticuloendothelial system and liver heparinase with approximately 50% urinary excretion of unchanged drug

protamine sulfate (1 mg neutralizes 90–115 units of heparin depending on preparation). Administer in a concentration of at least 10 mg/mL and bolus over 1–3 minutes. Do not exceed 50 mg in any 10-minute interval. There is no established role for dialysis

Dosing Information

Initial Loading Dose. 5000–10,000 units undiluted IV bolus. May repeat every 4–6 hours as necessary or initiate continuous infusion

Open Heart Surgery. 300–400 units/kg undiluted IV bolus and repeat as necessary to maintain ACT 400–600 seconds

DIC. 50–100 units/kg undiluted IV bolus—repeat every 4 hours as necessary but discontinue if no improvement in 4–8 hours

Initial Infusion Rate. 1000 units/hour

Maintenance Infusion Range. 800–1600 units/hour on average

Maximum Infusion Rate. Approximately 40,000 units/day

Titration Guideline

Suggested Regimen. Adjust dose such that activated PTT is 1.5–2.5 times control value or ACT is 2–3 times control value in seconds

Potential Drug Interactions

Potentiation of Heparin Effects. Warfarin, dextran, phenylbutazone, thrombolytic agents, salicylates, penicillins, cephalosporines, nonsteroidal anti-inflammatory agents, dihydroergotamine, dipyridamole

Antagonism of Heparin Effects. Intravenous nitroglycerin and possibly cardiac glycosides, nicotine, quinine, tetracycline

Possibly Antagonized by Heparin. Insulin, corticosteroids, corticotropin

Heparin Sodium

How Supplied

Parenteral Injection, Heparin Sodium
1000 units/mL—1-, 2-, 5-, 10-, and 30-mL vials
2500 units/mL—1-mL syringe
5000 units/mL—0.5-, 1-, and 10-mL vials
7500 units/mL—1-mL syringe
10,000 units/mL—0.5-, 1-, 4-, 5-, and 10-mL vials
20,000 units/mL—1-, 2-, 5-, and 10-mL vials
40,000 units/mL—1-, 2-, and 5-mL vials

Parenteral Injection, Heparin Calcium.

5000 units/mL—0.2-mL syringe

Premixed Infusion Bags—Heparin Sodium.

40 units/mL—50-mL (20,000 units) 5% dextrose injection

50 units/mL—250-mL (12,500) and 500-mL (25,000) 5% dextrose or 0.45% sodium chloride injection

100 units/mL—100-mL (10,000 units) 5% dextrose injection
250-mL (25,000 units) 5% dextrose or 0.45% sodium chloride injection

Principal Adverse Effects

CNS. Headache

Pulmonary. Asthma, tachypnea

CV. Chest pain, hypertension

GI. Nausea, vomiting

Heme. Hemorrhage at virtually any body site, including adrenal, ovarian, and retroperitoneal locations; thrombocytopenia; disseminated thrombotic syndromes (heparin-induced thrombocytopenia thrombosis)

Allergic. Peripheral vasospasm, urticaria, rhinitis, anaphylactoid reactions, shock

Miscellaneous. Chills, fever, cutaneous necrosis, aldosterone suppression, transient alopecia, priapism, rebound hyperlipidemia (high doses for long term), acute adrenal insufficiency, osteoporosis, decreased renal function

Heparin Sodium

20,000 units in 500 mL

■ Infusion Rate in mL/hr (pump setting) ■ Drug Dose in units/hr

mL/hr	units/hr	mL/hr	units/hr	mL/hr	units/hr	mL/hr	units/hr	mL/hr	units/hr	mL/hr	units/hr
1	40	21	840	41	1640	61	2440	81	3240	101	4040
2	80	22	880	42	1680	62	2480	82	3280	102	4080
3	120	23	920	43	1720	63	2520	83	3320	103	4120
4	160	24	960	44	1760	64	2560	84	3360	104	4160
5	200	25	1000	45	1800	65	2600	85	3400	105	4200
6	240	26	1040	46	1840	66	2640	86	3440	106	4240
7	280	27	1080	47	1880	67	2680	87	3480	107	4280
8	320	28	1120	48	1920	68	2720	88	3520	108	4320
9	360	29	1160	49	1960	69	2760	89	3560	109	4360
10	400	30	1200	50	2000	70	2800	90	3600	110	4400
11	440	31	1240	51	2040	71	2840	91	3640	111	4440
12	480	32	1280	52	2080	72	2880	92	3680	112	4480
13	520	33	1320	53	2120	73	2920	93	3720	113	4520
14	560	34	1360	54	2160	74	2960	94	3760	114	4560
15	600	35	1400	55	2200	75	3000	95	3800	115	4600
16	640	36	1440	56	2240	76	3040	96	3840	116	4640
17	680	37	1480	57	2280	77	3080	97	3880	117	4680
18	720	38	1520	58	2320	78	3120	98	3920	118	4720
19	760	39	1560	59	2360	79	3160	99	3860	119	4760
20	800	40	1600	60	2400	80	3200	100	4000	120	4800

■ Infusion Rate in mL/hr (pump setting) ■ Drug Dose in units/hr

mL/hr	units/hr	mL/hr	units/hr	mL/hr	units/hr	mL/hr	units/hr	mL/hr	units/hr	mL/hr	units/hr
1	100	21	2100	41	4100	61	6100	81	8100	101	10100
2	200	22	2200	42	4200	62	6200	82	8200	102	10200
3	300	23	2300	43	4300	63	6300	83	8300	103	10300
4	400	24	2400	44	4400	64	6400	84	8400	104	10400
5	500	25	2500	45	4500	65	6500	85	8500	105	10500
6	600	26	2600	46	4600	66	6600	86	8600	106	10600
7	700	27	2700	47	4700	67	6700	87	8700	107	10700
8	800	28	2800	48	4800	68	6800	88	8800	108	10800
9	900	29	2900	49	4900	69	6900	89	8900	109	10900
10	1000	30	3000	50	5000	70	7000	90	9000	110	11000
11	1100	31	3100	51	5100	71	7100	91	9100	111	11100
12	1200	32	3200	52	5200	72	7200	92	9200	112	11200
13	1300	33	3300	53	5300	73	7300	93	9300	113	11300
14	1400	34	3400	54	5400	74	7400	94	9400	114	11400
15	1500	35	3500	55	5500	75	7500	95	9500	115	11500
16	1600	36	3600	56	5600	76	7600	96	9600	116	11600
17	1700	37	3700	57	5700	77	7700	97	9700	117	11700
18	1800	38	3800	58	5800	78	7800	98	9800	118	11800
19	1900	39	3900	59	5900	79	7900	99	9900	119	11900
20	2000	40	4000	60	6000	80	8000	100	10000	120	12000

Insulin (Regular)

Pharmacology

Endogenous hormone secreted by beta cells of the pancreas—may be synthetically produced by recombinant DNA technology

Facilitates transport of glucose into myocytes and adipocytes and enhances liver phosphorylation of glucose to glucose-6-phosphate

Stimulates protein synthesis, carbohydrate metabolism, and lipogenesis

Inhibits lipolysis and free fatty acid release from the adipocytes

May temporarily decrease serum potassium and magnesium levels causing intracellular shifts of these cations

Enables type I diabetics to convert glycogen to fat; store glucose in the liver; and metabolize carbohydrates, proteins, and fats

Administrative Guidelines

Administer infusion via precision control device

Frequently monitor serum glucose concentrations and electrolytes, particularly potassium and magnesium; carefully follow vital signs and ECG

For infusion, recommend diluting with 0.9% sodium chloride solution

After serum glucose levels are initially controlled, infusion of dextrose solutions may be needed to prevent hypoglycemia

Electrolyte replacement therapy may be necessary

After addition to an IV infusion solution, actual dose delivered to patient may be reduced by 20% to 80% owing to absorption of insulin by the container and tubing

When mixing regular with other insulin preparations, first draw regular insulin into syringe to avoid contamination of the regular insulin vial; administer

(continued below)

Indications

Emergency treatment of diabetic coma or ketoacidosis

Initial therapy of type I diabetes mellitus when rapid control of serum glucose is necessary

Management of type II diabetic patients with inadequate glucose control associated with endocrine disorders, surgery, pregnancy, fever, sepsis, trauma, or other major illnesses

Control of severe hypokalemia in conjunction with IV dextrose solution

Diagnostic evaluation of pituitary growth hormone reserve in patients with suspected or known growth hormone deficiency

mixture immediately because binding of regular insulin by the other preparation occurs and results in a reduction of delivered dose

May need to reduce dose in patients with adrenocortical insufficiency

Insulin resistance may develop because of obesity-induced tissue insensitivity or formation of antibodies or in patients with emotional disturbances, surgery, trauma, infections, or additional endocrine disorders. Consider changing from beef to pork preparations (or vice versa) or to a purified preparation and treating the concurrent medical illness

Contraindicated in patients with known hypersensitivity

Use cautiously in patients with renal impairment, adrenal insufficiency, or those receiving propranolol

Overdosage leads to hypoglycemia, which may cause psychiatric disturbances, such as mania, aphasia, or changes in personality, and lead to irreversible brain damage. Symptoms of hypoglycemia include

(continued on page 124)

Insulin (Regular)

Pharmacokinetics

Onset of Action. 30 minutes–1 hour

Peak Effects. 2–3 hours

Duration of Action. 5–7 hours

Plasma Half-Life. Few minutes in healthy patients, but up to 13 hours in diabetics (probably owing to presence of insulin antibodies)

Metabolism. Via liver with filtering at the glomerulus and reabsorption at the proximal tubule

diaphoresis, headache, fatigue, pallor, nausea, palpitations, paresthesias, tremors, visual changes, hyperthermia, mental confusion, seizures, and loss of consciousness. Manage with oral carbohydrates for mild reactions and 10–30 mL of a 50% dextrose solution IV for severe reactions or coma

Dosing Information

Initial Loading Dose for Diabetic Ketoacidosis. 0.1 units/kg IV bolus (or 2.4–7.2 units IV bolus)

Maintenance Infusion Range. 0.1–0.2 units/kg/hour (or 2.4 to 7.2 units/hour)

Maximum Infusion Rate. 0.2 units/kg/hour

Severe Ketoacidosis with Coma. 50–100 units IV bolus with equal amounts given simultaneously subcutaneously. Subsequent doses every 1–2 hours as necessary based on blood glucose, acetone, ketone measurements, and patient response

Severe Ketoacidosis with Circulatory Collapse. 100–200 units IV bolus. Subsequent doses every 1–2 hours as necessary based on blood glucose, acetone, ketone measurements, and clinical response

Titration Guideline for Ketoacidosis. Adjust infusion by 0.05 units/hour as required for serum glucose control

(continued on page 126)

Potential Drug Interactions

Potentiation of Insulin Effects. Salicylates, anabolic steroids, alcohol, monoamine oxidase inhibitors, guanethidine, propranolol

Antagonism of Insulin Effects. Epinephrine, corticosteroids, oral contraceptives, thiazides, furosemide, ethacrynic acid, diazoxide, phenytoin, somatotropin, estrogens, thyroid hormones

Insulin (Regular)

Moderate to Severe Hyperkalemia. 10 units IV bolus concurrent with 200–500 mL of 10% dextrose solution USP over 30 minutes, followed by 500–1000 mL over the next several hours

Growth Hormone Reserve. 0.05–0.15 units/kg rapid IV injection

How Supplied

40 units/mL—beef and pork in 10-mL bottle of 400 units

100 units/mL—pork in 10-mL vials of 1000 units
purified pork in 10-mL bottles and vials of 1000 units
purified beef in 10-mL bottles of 1000 units
human insulin (rDNA) in 10-mL bottles of 1000 units
buffered human insulin (rDNA) in 10-mL bottles of 1000 units
human insulin semisynthetic in 10-mL bottles of 1000 units

Principal Adverse Effects

CNS. Aphasia, mania, personality changes, headache, confusion, paresthesias, tremor, seizures, coma, loss of consciousness, yawning, muscle weakness, fatigue, irritability

Respiratory. Shallow breathing

CV. Tachycardia, palpitations

GI. Hunger, nausea

Allergic. Urticaria, lymphadenopathy, angioedema, anaphylaxis

Miscellaneous. Visual disturbances, hypothermia, diaphoresis, pallor, perioral numbness, Somogyi responses (hyperglycemic rebound)

Insulin (Regular)

200 units in 1000 mL

■ Infusion Rate in mL/hr (pump setting) ■ Drug Dose in units/hr

mL/hr	units/hr	mL/hr	units/hr	mL/hr	units/hr	mL/hr	units/hr	mL/hr	units/hr	mL/hr	units/hr
1	0.2	21	4.2	41	8.2	61	12.2	81	16.2	101	20.2
2	0.4	22	4.4	42	8.4	62	12.4	82	16.4	102	20.4
3	0.6	23	4.6	43	8.6	63	12.6	83	16.6	103	20.6
4	0.8	24	4.8	44	8.8	64	12.8	84	16.8	104	20.8
5	1.0	25	5.0	45	9.0	65	13.0	85	17.0	105	21.0
6	1.2	26	5.2	46	9.2	66	13.2	86	17.2	106	21.2
7	1.4	27	5.4	47	9.4	67	13.4	87	17.4	107	21.4
8	1.6	28	5.6	48	9.6	68	13.6	88	17.6	108	21.6
9	1.8	29	5.8	49	9.8	69	13.8	89	17.8	109	21.8
10	2.0	30	6.0	50	10.0	70	14.0	90	18.0	110	22.0
11	2.2	31	6.2	51	10.2	71	14.2	91	18.2	111	22.2
12	2.4	32	6.4	52	10.4	72	14.4	92	18.4	112	22.4
13	2.6	33	6.6	53	10.6	73	14.6	93	18.6	113	22.6
14	2.8	34	6.8	54	10.8	74	14.8	94	18.8	114	22.8
15	3.0	35	7.0	55	11.0	75	15.0	95	19.0	115	23.0
16	3.2	36	7.2	56	11.2	76	15.2	96	19.2	116	23.2
17	3.4	37	7.4	57	11.4	77	15.4	97	19.4	117	23.4
18	3.6	38	7.6	58	11.6	78	15.6	98	19.6	118	23.6
19	3.8	39	7.8	59	11.8	79	15.8	99	19.8	119	23.8
20	4.0	40	8.0	60	12.0	80	16.0	100	20.0	120	24.0

DRUG DOSE in units/kg/hr

Infusion Rate in mL/hr	Patient's Weight kg 40 / lbs 88	45 / 99	50 / 110	55 / 121	60 / 132	65 / 143	70 / 154	75 / 165	80 / 176	85 / 187	90 / 198	95 / 209	100 / 220	105 / 231	110 / 242
5	0.025	0.022	0.020	0.018	0.017	0.015	0.014	0.013	0.013	0.012	0.011	0.011	0.010	0.010	0.009
10	0.050	0.044	0.040	0.036	0.033	0.031	0.029	0.027	0.025	0.024	0.022	0.021	0.020	0.019	0.018
15	0.075	0.067	0.060	0.055	0.050	0.046	0.043	0.040	0.038	0.035	0.033	0.032	0.030	0.029	0.027
20	0.100	0.089	0.080	0.073	0.067	0.062	0.057	0.053	0.050	0.047	0.044	0.042	0.040	0.038	0.036
25	0.125	0.111	0.100	0.091	0.083	0.077	0.071	0.067	0.063	0.059	0.056	0.053	0.050	0.048	0.045
30	0.150	0.133	0.120	0.109	0.100	0.092	0.086	0.080	0.075	0.071	0.067	0.063	0.060	0.057	0.055
35	0.175	0.156	0.140	0.127	0.117	0.108	0.100	0.093	0.087	0.082	0.078	0.074	0.070	0.067	0.064
40	0.200	0.178	0.160	0.145	0.133	0.123	0.114	0.107	0.100	0.094	0.089	0.084	0.080	0.076	0.073
45	0.225	0.200	0.180	0.164	0.150	0.138	0.129	0.120	0.112	0.106	0.100	0.095	0.090	0.086	0.082
50	0.250	0.222	0.200	0.182	0.167	0.154	0.143	0.133	0.125	0.118	0.111	0.105	0.100	0.095	0.091
55	0.275	0.244	0.220	0.200	0.183	0.169	0.157	0.147	0.138	0.129	0.122	0.116	0.110	0.105	0.100
60	0.300	0.267	0.240	0.218	0.200	0.185	0.171	0.160	0.150	0.141	0.133	0.126	0.120	0.114	0.109
65	0.325	0.289	0.260	0.236	0.217	0.200	0.186	0.173	0.162	0.153	0.144	0.137	0.130	0.124	0.118
70	0.350	0.311	0.280	0.255	0.233	0.215	0.200	0.187	0.175	0.165	0.156	0.147	0.140	0.133	0.127
75	0.375	0.333	0.300	0.273	0.250	0.231	0.214	0.200	0.188	0.176	0.167	0.158	0.150	0.143	0.136
80	0.400	0.356	0.320	0.291	0.267	0.246	0.229	0.213	0.200	0.188	0.178	0.168	0.160	0.152	0.145
85	0.425	0.378	0.340	0.309	0.283	0.262	0.243	0.227	0.213	0.200	0.189	0.179	0.170	0.162	0.155
90	0.450	0.400	0.360	0.327	0.300	0.277	0.257	0.240	0.225	0.212	0.200	0.189	0.180	0.171	0.164
95	0.475	0.422	0.380	0.345	0.317	0.292	0.271	0.253	0.237	0.224	0.211	0.200	0.190	0.181	0.173
100	0.500	0.444	0.400	0.364	0.333	0.308	0.286	0.267	0.250	0.235	0.222	0.211	0.200	0.190	0.182
105	0.525	0.467	0.420	0.382	0.350	0.323	0.300	0.280	0.262	0.247	0.233	0.221	0.210	0.200	0.191
110	0.550	0.489	0.440	0.400	0.367	0.338	0.314	0.293	0.275	0.259	0.244	0.232	0.220	0.210	0.200
115	0.575	0.511	0.460	0.418	0.383	0.354	0.329	0.307	0.287	0.271	0.256	0.242	0.230	0.219	0.209
120	0.600	0.533	0.480	0.436	0.400	0.369	0.343	0.320	0.300	0.282	0.267	0.253	0.240	0.229	0.218

Isoproterenol Hydrochloride (Isuprel)

Pharmacology

Synthetic sympathomimetic agent that acts directly on beta-adrenergic receptors—no significant alpha-adrenergic effects

Mechanism of action presumed to be activation of adenyl cyclase with cyclic AMP production

Produces chronotropic and inotropic ($beta_1$) cardiac effects, which usually increase systolic blood pressure, heart rate, coronary artery blood flow, cardiac output, and myocardial oxygen consumption

May potentiate myocardial ischemia via direct coronary vasodilation and production of coronary steal syndrome

Shortens conduction time and refractory period of the atrioventricular node in atrioventricular block

Relaxation of smooth muscle ($beta_2$) effects predominantly in the gastrointestinal tract, bronchial tree, and uterus

(continued below)

Administrative Guidelines

Administer infusion via precision control device

Continuously monitor ECG and blood pressure; carefully follow hemodynamic variables, acid-base status, renal function, and electrolytes

Correct hypovolemia and acid-base and metabolic abnormalities, if possible, before and during administration

Discontinue infusion immediately if precordial discomfort, angina, or ventricular dysrhythmias occur

Excessive tachycardia (heart rate ≥110) requires reduction or temporary discontinuation of infusion

May cause tachyphylaxis with prolonged or frequent use

Contraindicated with known hypersensitivity, digitalis toxicity, preexisting tachydysrhythmias, and angina pectoris

(continued below)

Vasodilates peripheral arterioles (beta$_2$ effect) in skeletal muscle, pulmonary, mesenteric, and intestinal vascular sites

Variable effects on renal blood flow and lactic acid production

Inhibits release of histamine and slow-reacting substance of anaphylaxis

Increases liver glycogenolysis, serum free fatty acids, and insulin release

Indications

Adjunctive treatment for low cardiac output states and shock syndromes, especially characterized by peripheral vasoconstriction (generally avoid use with acute myocardial infarction)

Treatment of refractory bradydysrhythmias and carotid sinus hypersensitivity

Unlabeled Uses. Pulmonary embolism, torsades de pointes, and as a diagnostic aid in detecting coronary artery disease

Use with caution in geriatric patients; those with diabetes mellitus, hyperthyroidism, angina pectoris and acute coronary syndromes, hypotension, hypovolemia, or renal disease; those taking digitalis or diuretics; and those with known sensitivity to sympathomimetics

Overdosage may manifest with blood pressure disturbances, palpitations, angina, tachycardia, or other dysrhythmias. Manage with general supportive measures coincident with termination of infusion

Isoproterenol Hydrochloride (Isuprel)

Pharmacokinetics

Onset of Action. Immediate

Peak Effects. Within 15 minutes

Duration of Action. Less than 1 hour (8–50 minutes)

Metabolism. Principally via the gastrointestinal tract and liver with urinary excretion

Dosing Information

IV Bolus Dose for Dysrhythmias. 20–60 μg (1–3 mL of ***1:50,000*** solution) initially; 10–200 μg (0.5–10 mL of ***1:50,000*** solution) thereafter as necessary

Initial Infusion Rate. 0.5 μg/min

Maintenance Infusion Range. 0.5–10 μg/min

Maximum Infusion Rate. 30 μg/min except in severe shock syndromes

Titration Guideline

Suggested Regimen. Adjust infusion by 0.5–2 μg/min every 5–15 minutes as required

How Supplied

1:5000 (200 μg/mL)—1-mL ampuls of 200 μg
5-mL ampuls and vials of 1000 μg
10-mL vials of 2000 μg

1:50,000 (20 μg/mL)—1-mL ampuls of 20 μg

Potential Drug Interactions

Potentiation of Isoproterenol Effects. Digitalis, theophyllines, epinephrine, cyclopropane or halogenated hydrocarbon anesthetics, oxytocic agents, monoamine oxidase inhibitors, tricyclic antidepressants, guanethidine, bretylium

Antagonism of Isoproterenol Effects. Beta-blockers

Principal Adverse Effects

CNS. Dizziness, weakness, headache, nervousness, sweating, flushing, tremors, tinnitus, insomnia, anxiety, fear, excitement, asthenia

Pulmonary. Isolated report of pulmonary edema

CV. Palpitations, angina, tachydysrhythmias, Stokes-Adams attacks, heart block, hypertension, hypotension, shock, focal myocardial necrosis

GI. Nausea and vomiting

Miscellaneous. Parotid gland swelling

Isoproterenol Hydrochloride (Isuprel) 3 mg in 250 mL

■ Infusion Rate in mL/hr (pump setting) ■ Drug Dose in μg/min

mL/hr	μg/min	mL/hr	μg/min	mL/hr	μg/min	mL/hr	μg/min	mL/hr	μg/min	mL/hr	μg/min
1	0.2	21	4.2	41	8.2	61	12.2	81	16.2	101	20.2
2	0.4	22	4.4	42	8.4	62	12.4	82	16.4	102	20.4
3	0.6	23	4.6	43	8.6	63	12.6	83	16.6	103	20.6
4	0.8	24	4.8	44	8.8	64	12.8	84	16.8	104	20.8
5	1.0	25	5.0	45	9.0	65	13.0	85	17.0	105	21.0
6	1.2	26	5.2	46	9.2	66	13.2	86	17.2	106	21.2
7	1.4	27	5.4	47	9.4	67	13.4	87	17.4	107	21.4
8	1.6	28	5.6	48	9.6	68	13.6	88	17.6	108	21.6
9	1.8	29	5.8	49	9.8	69	13.8	89	17.8	109	21.8
10	2.0	30	6.0	50	10.0	70	14.0	90	18.0	110	22.0
11	2.2	31	6.2	51	10.2	71	14.2	91	18.2	111	22.2
12	2.4	32	6.4	52	10.4	72	14.4	92	18.4	112	22.4
13	2.6	33	6.6	53	10.6	73	14.6	93	18.6	113	22.6
14	2.8	34	6.8	54	10.8	74	14.8	94	18.8	114	22.8
15	3.0	35	7.0	55	11.0	75	15.0	95	19.0	115	23.0
16	3.2	36	7.2	56	11.2	76	15.2	96	19.2	116	23.2
17	3.4	37	7.4	57	11.4	77	15.4	97	19.4	117	23.4
18	3.6	38	7.6	58	11.6	78	15.6	98	19.6	118	23.6
19	3.8	39	7.8	59	11.8	79	15.8	99	19.8	119	23.8
20	4.0	40	8.0	60	12.0	80	16.0	100	20.0	120	24.0

Isoproterenol Hydrochloride (Isuprel) 6 mg in 250 mL

■ **Infusion Rate in mL/hr (pump setting)** ■ **Drug Dose in μg/min**

mL/hr	μg/min	mL/hr	μg/min	mL/hr	μg/min	mL/hr	μg/min	mL/hr	μg/min	mL/hr	μg/min
1	0.4	21	8.4	41	16.4	61	24.4	81	32.4	101	40.4
2	0.8	22	8.8	42	16.8	62	24.8	82	32.8	102	40.8
3	1.2	23	9.2	43	17.2	63	25.2	83	33.2	103	41.2
4	1.6	24	9.6	44	17.6	64	25.6	84	33.6	104	41.6
5	2.0	25	10.0	45	18.0	65	26.0	85	34.0	105	42.0
6	2.4	26	10.4	46	18.4	66	26.4	86	34.4	106	42.4
7	2.8	27	10.8	47	18.8	67	26.8	87	34.8	107	42.8
8	3.2	28	11.2	48	19.2	68	27.2	88	35.2	108	43.2
9	3.6	29	11.6	49	19.6	69	27.6	89	35.6	109	43.6
10	4.0	30	12.0	50	20.0	70	28.0	90	36.0	110	44.0
11	4.4	31	12.4	51	20.4	71	28.4	91	36.4	111	44.4
12	4.8	32	12.8	52	20.8	72	28.8	92	36.8	112	44.8
13	5.2	33	13.2	53	21.2	73	29.2	93	37.2	113	45.2
14	5.6	34	13.6	54	21.6	74	29.6	94	37.6	114	45.6
15	6.0	35	14.0	55	22.0	75	30.0	95	38.0	115	46.0
16	6.4	36	14.4	56	22.4	76	30.4	96	38.4	116	46.4
17	6.8	37	14.8	57	22.8	77	30.8	97	38.8	117	46.8
18	7.2	38	15.2	58	23.2	78	31.2	98	39.2	118	47.2
19	7.6	39	15.6	59	23.6	79	31.6	99	39.6	119	47.6
20	8.0	40	16.0	60	24.0	80	32.0	100	40.0	120	48.0

Labetalol Hydrochloride (Normodyne)

Pharmacology

Competitively blocks alpha$_1$-receptors in vascular smooth muscle, beta$_1$-receptors in the heart, and beta$_2$-receptors in bronchial and vascular smooth muscle

Produces dose-dependent reduction in blood pressure and systemic vascular resistance potentiated by standing

No significant effects on heart rate, cardiac output, or stroke volume unless coronary artery disease is present (may decrease these parameters as well as blood pressure if coronary artery disease present)

May decrease atrioventricular node conduction velocity and prolong atrial effective refractory period

No significant reduction in cerebral blood flow, renal blood flow, or glomerular filtration rate

May decrease plasma aldosterone and angiotensin II levels

May increase airway resistance

May increase plasma glucose and prolactin levels

Administrative Guidelines

Administer infusion via precision control device

Carefully monitor blood pressure at 5-minute intervals before and during infusion

Always maintain patients in supine position during infusion

Following discontinuation of IV therapy, monitor blood pressure at 5-minute intervals for 30 minutes, then 30-minute intervals for 2 hours, then hourly for 6 hours, then as necessary

Begin oral therapy when supine diastolic pressure has increased by 10 mmHg

Patients should remain supine for at least 3 hours following drug discontinuation

Contraindicated in patients with overt heart failure, bronchial asthma, second-degree or third-degree block, cardiogenic shock, severe bradycardia, severe hypotension, and known hypersensitivity

(continued below)

Indications

Management of hypertension and hypertensive emergencies

Unlabeled uses. Prevention and treatment of clonidine withdrawal syndromes, during anesthesia or laryngoscopy, for stable angina and sympathetic overactivity associated with tetanus

Pharmacokinetics

Onset of Action. 2–5 minutes

Peak Effects. 5–15 minutes

Duration of Action. 2–4 hours but rarely up to 24 hours

Elimination Half-Life. 2.5–8 hours

Metabolism. Via liver with urinary, biliary, and fecal elimination

Use with caution in those with depressed cardiac function, pheochromocytoma, diabetics on hypoglycemic therapy, with halothane anesthesia and general surgery, impaired hepatic function, and those receiving other hypotensive agents

Overdosage requires specific supportive measures. Consider 5–10 mg IV glucagon followed by 5 mg/hour for severe beta-blocker toxicity. Dialysis is not effective

Labetalol Hydrochloride (Normodyne)

Dosing Information

Initial IV Bolus Dose. 20 mg over 2 minutes. May repeat 20–80 mg IV bolus at 10-minute intervals as necessary

Maximal IV Bolus Dose. 1–2 mg/kg

Initial IV Infusion Dose. 2 mg/min

Alternative IV Infusion Regimen. 20 mg/hour for 1 hour, then 40 mg/hour for 1 hour, then 80 mg/hour for 1 hour, then 160 mg/hour as necessary

Maximum Cumulative Dose. 300 mg

Titration Guideline

Suggested Regimen. Adjust infusion by 1–2 mg/min as necessary for effective blood pressure control

How Supplied

5 mg/mL—20-mL ampuls and multidose vials of 100 mg
40-mL multidose vials of 200 mg
60-mL multidose vials of 300 mg

Potential Drug Interactions

Potentiation of Labetalol Effects. Diuretics and other hypotensive agents, beta-blockers, calcium channel blockers, halothane, cimetidine, nitroglycerin

Antagonism of Labetalol Effects. Glutethimide, $beta_1$ and $beta_2$ agonists, alpha agonists

Possibly Antagonized by Labetalol. Bronchodilators

Principal Adverse Effects

CNS. Dizziness, vertigo, scalp tingling, numbness, yawning, somnolence, mental depression, disorientation

CV. Ventricular dysrhythmias, postural hypotension, atrioventricular block, bradycardia, chest pain, heart failure, syncope

GI. Dyspepsia, taste distortion, nausea, vomiting

Renal. Transient increases in BUN and creatinine

Miscellaneous. Wheezing, flushing, pruritus, diaphoresis, interference with plasma catecholamine determinations, anaphylactoid reactions

Labetalol Hydrochloride (Normodyne) 200 mg in 200 mL

■ Infusion Rate in mL/hr (pump setting) ■ Drug Dose in mg/min

mL/hr	mg/min	mL/hr	mg/min	mL/hr	mg/min	mL/hr	mg/min	mL/hr	mg/min	mL/hr	mg/min
1	0.02	21	0.35	41	0.68	61	1.02	81	1.35	101	1.68
2	0.03	22	0.37	42	0.70	62	1.03	82	1.37	102	1.70
3	0.05	23	0.38	43	0.72	63	1.05	83	1.38	103	1.72
4	0.07	24	0.40	44	0.73	64	1.07	84	1.40	104	1.73
5	0.08	25	0.42	45	0.75	65	1.08	85	1.42	105	1.75
6	0.10	26	0.43	46	0.77	66	1.10	86	1.43	106	1.77
7	0.12	27	0.45	47	0.78	67	1.12	87	1.45	107	1.78
8	0.13	28	0.47	48	0.80	68	1.13	88	1.47	108	1.80
9	0.15	29	0.48	49	0.82	69	1.15	89	1.48	109	1.82
10	0.17	30	0.50	50	0.83	70	1.17	90	1.50	110	1.83
11	0.18	31	0.52	51	0.85	71	1.18	91	1.52	111	1.85
12	0.20	32	0.53	52	0.87	72	1.20	92	1.53	112	1.87
13	0.22	33	0.55	53	0.88	73	1.22	93	1.55	113	1.88
14	0.23	34	0.57	54	0.90	74	1.23	94	1.57	114	1.90
15	0.25	35	0.58	55	0.92	75	1.25	95	1.58	115	1.92
16	0.27	36	0.60	56	0.93	76	1.27	96	1.60	116	1.93
17	0.28	37	0.62	57	0.95	77	1.28	97	1.62	117	1.95
18	0.30	38	0.63	58	0.97	78	1.30	98	1.63	118	1.97
19	0.32	39	0.65	59	0.98	79	1.32	99	1.65	119	1.98
20	0.33	40	0.67	60	1.00	80	1.33	100	1.67	120	2.00

Labetalol Hydrochloride (Normodyne) 600 mg in 250 mL

■ Infusion Rate in mL/hr (pump setting) ■ Drug Dose in mg/min

mL/hr	mg/min	mL/hr	mg/min	mL/hr	mg/min	mL/hr	mg/min	mL/hr	mg/min	mL/hr	mg/min
1	0.04	21	0.84	41	1.64	61	2.44	81	3.24	101	4.04
2	0.08	22	0.88	42	1.68	62	2.48	82	3.28	102	4.08
3	0.12	23	0.92	43	1.72	63	2.52	83	3.30	103	4.12
4	0.16	24	0.96	44	1.76	64	2.56	84	3.36	104	4.16
5	0.20	25	1.00	45	1.80	65	2.60	85	3.40	105	4.20
6	0.24	26	1.04	46	1.84	66	2.64	86	3.44	106	4.24
7	0.28	27	1.08	47	1.88	67	2.68	87	3.48	107	4.28
8	0.32	28	1.12	48	1.92	68	2.72	88	3.52	108	4.32
9	0.36	29	1.16	49	1.96	69	2.76	89	3.56	109	4.36
10	0.40	30	1.20	50	2.00	70	2.80	90	3.60	110	4.40
11	0.44	31	1.24	51	2.04	71	2.84	91	3.64	111	4.44
12	0.48	32	1.28	52	2.08	72	2.88	92	3.68	112	4.48
13	0.52	33	1.32	53	2.12	73	2.92	93	3.72	113	4.52
14	0.56	34	1.36	54	2.16	74	2.96	94	3.76	114	4.56
15	0.60	35	1.40	55	2.20	75	3.00	95	3.80	115	4.60
16	0.64	36	1.44	56	2.24	76	3.04	96	3.84	116	4.64
17	0.60	37	1.48	57	2.28	77	3.08	97	3.88	117	4.68
18	0.70	38	1.52	58	2.32	78	3.12	98	3.92	118	4.72
19	0.76	39	1.56	59	2.36	79	3.16	99	3.96	119	4.76
20	0.80	40	1.60	60	2.40	80	3.20	100	4.00	120	4.80

Lidocaine Hydrochloride (Xylocaine)

Pharmacology

Vaughn-Williams class IB antiarrhythmic with local anesthetic properties

Stabilizes cell membranes by interacting with fast sodium channels in a time-dependent and voltage-dependent manner

Electrophysiological effects include suppressing His-Purkinje automaticity and phase 4 diastolic depolarization of the ventricles. Also decreases action potential duration and effective refractory period of Purkinje fibers and ventricular muscle—no effect on excitability of cardiac tissue

Raises ventricular fibrillation threshold. No significant atrial, sinoatrial nodal, autonomic, or myocardial depressant effects

May decrease heart rate and atrioventricular conduction in patients with preexisting sinoatrial or atrioventricular node disease

May increase coronary blood flow

(continued below)

Administrative Guidelines

Administer infusion via precision control device

Continuously monitor ECG and carefully follow serum electrolytes, magnesium, calcium, and acid-base status

Correct metabolic abnormalities and hypoxia, if possible, before use

Monitor serum drug levels, especially if toxicity suspected

May be given via endotracheal tube. Use 2–2.5 times the IV dose and dilute with 10 mL of distilled water or normal saline

Reduce dose or discontinue infusion if excessive prolongation of PR or QRS intervals noted or new dysrhythmias appear

Contraindicated in patients with known hypersensitivity; Stokes-Adams syndrome; or severe sinoatrial node, atrioventricular node, or intraventricular block without a functioning artificial pacemaker

(continued below)

CNS depressant with sedative, analgesic, and anticonvulsant actions—suppresses cough and gag reflexes

Indications

Acute prophylaxis and treatment of ventricular dysrhythmias

Pharmacokinetics

Onset of Action. 45–90 seconds

Peak Effects. 1–2 minutes

Duration of Action. 10–30 minutes after IV bolus

IV Bolus (Distribution) Half-Life. 7–30 minutes

IV Infusion (Elimination) Half-Life. 90–120 minutes. May be prolonged after 24–48 hour infusion in heart and liver failure and with acute myocardial infarction

Metabolism. Via liver with urinary excretion

Use with Caution in patients with atrial fibrillation, Wolff-Parkinson-White syndrome, bradycardia, heart block, excessive QRS prolongation, severe respiratory depression, hypovolemia, shock, liver disease, renal disease, hypoxia, congestive heart failure, CNS disturbances, and those predisposed to malignant hyperthermia

Overdosage may manifest with CNS disturbances, including seizures. Dysrhythmias, hypotension, and cardiovascular collapse may also occur. Manage with emergency resuscitative and supportive measures. Consider diazepam or thiopental for seizures and vasopressors for severe hypotension. There is no established role for dialysis

Lidocaine Hydrochloride (Xylocaine)

Dosing Information

IV Bolus Dose for Cardiac Arrest. 1.0–1.5 mg/kg over 1–2 minutes. May repeat 0.5–1.5 mg/kg IV bolus at 5–10 minute intervals as necessary up to 3 mg/kg

Initial IV Loading Dose for Dysrhythmias. 50–100 mg undiluted bolus over 1–2 minutes, then 50-mg boluses every 5 minutes × 3

Maintenance Infusion Range. 1–4 mg/min

Maximum Infusion Rate. 4 mg/min

Consider reduced loading dose or infusion rate in the elderly, those with heart failure, and those with liver disease. Do not administer more than 300 mg in any 1-hour period

Therapeutic Level

1.5–6.0 μg/mL

Potential Drug Interactions

Potentiation of Lidocaine Effects. Cimetidine, phenytoin, procainamide, propranolol and other beta-blockers, tubocurarine, quinidine, tocainide, mexiletine, neomycin, polymyxin B

Possibly Potentiated by Lidocaine. Succinylcholine

Principal Adverse Effects

CNS. Respiratory depression, drowsiness, apprehension, visual disturbances, tremors, paresthesias, lightheadedness, tinnitus, seizures, coma, psychosis, euphoria, and other idiosyncratic reactions

Pulmonary. Dyspnea, respiratory depression and arrest

(continued below)

Titration Guideline

Suggested Regimen. 0.5 mg/kg undiluted IV bolus followed by 1 mg/min increase in infusion rate as required for dysrhythmia control. Omission of bolus delays new steady-state from being achieved for 5–8 hours

How Supplied

IV Bolus Use

10 mg/mL (1%)—5-mL ampuls and syringes of 50 mg
vials of 20 mL (200 mg), 30 mL (300 mg), and 50 mL(500 mg)

20 mg/mL (2%)—5-mL vials, ampuls, and syringes of 100 mg
vials of 10 mL (200 mg), 20 mL (400 mg), 30 mL (600 mg), and 50 mL (1000 mg)

(continued on page 146)

CV. Hypotension, bradycardia, dysrhythmias, heart block, cardiac arrest

GI. Dysphagia, nausea, vomiting

Allergic. Hypersensitivity reactions, edema, urticaria

Dermatological. Thrombophlebitis at infusion site

Miscellaneous. Malignant hyperthermia, fever

Lidocaine Hydrochloride (Xylocaine)

IV Admixture Use

40 mg/mL (4%)—5-mL ampuls of 200 mg
25-mL (1000 mg) vials and syringes
50-mL (2000 mg) vials and syringes

100 mg/mL (10%)—10-mL vials of 1000 mg

200 mg/mL (20%)—5-mL vials and syringes of 100 mg
10-mL vials and syringes of 2000 mg

IV Infusion Premixed

2 mg/mL (0.2%)—500 and 1000 mL 5% dextrose

4 mg/mL (0.4%)—250 and 500 mL 5% dextrose

8 mg/mL (0.8%)—250 and 500 mL 5% dextrose

Lidocaine Hydrochloride (Xylocaine) 2 g in 500 mL

■ Infusion Rate in mL/hr (pump setting) ■ Drug Dose in mg/min

mL/hr	mg/min	mL/hr	mg/min	mL/hr	mg/min	mL/hr	mg/min	mL/hr	mg/min	mL/hr	mg/min
1	0.07	21	1.40	41	2.73	61	4.07	81	5.40	101	6.73
2	0.13	22	1.47	42	2.80	62	4.13	82	5.47	102	6.80
3	0.20	23	1.53	43	2.87	63	4.20	83	5.53	103	6.87
4	0.27	24	1.60	44	2.93	64	4.27	84	5.60	104	6.93
5	0.33	25	1.67	45	3.00	65	4.33	85	5.67	105	7.00
6	0.40	26	1.73	46	3.07	66	4.40	86	5.73	106	7.07
7	0.47	27	1.80	47	3.13	67	4.47	87	5.80	107	7.13
8	0.53	28	1.87	48	3.20	68	4.53	88	5.87	108	7.20
9	0.60	29	1.93	49	3.27	69	4.60	89	5.93	109	7.27
10	0.67	30	2.00	50	3.33	70	4.67	90	6.00	110	7.33
11	0.73	31	2.07	51	3.40	71	4.73	91	6.07	111	7.40
12	0.80	32	2.13	52	3.47	72	4.80	92	6.13	112	7.47
13	0.87	33	2.20	53	3.53	73	4.87	93	6.20	113	7.53
14	0.93	34	2.27	54	3.60	74	4.93	94	6.27	114	7.60
15	1.00	35	2.33	55	3.67	75	5.00	95	6.33	115	7.67
16	1.07	36	2.40	56	3.73	76	5.07	96	6.40	116	7.73
17	1.13	37	2.47	57	3.80	77	5.13	97	6.47	117	7.80
18	1.20	38	2.53	58	3.87	78	5.20	98	6.53	118	7.87
19	1.27	39	2.60	59	3.93	79	5.27	99	6.60	119	7.93
20	1.33	40	2.67	60	4.00	80	5.33	100	6.67	120	8.00

■ Infusion Rate in mL/hr (pump setting) ■ Drug Dose in mg/min

mL/hr	mg/min	mL/hr	mg/min	mL/hr	mg/min	mL/hr	mg/min	mL/hr	mg/min	mL/hr	mg/min
1	0.13	21	2.80	41	5.47	61	8.13	81	10.80	101	13.47
2	0.27	22	2.93	42	5.60	62	8.27	82	10.93	102	13.60
3	0.40	23	3.07	43	5.73	63	8.40	83	11.07	103	13.73
4	0.53	24	3.20	44	5.87	64	8.53	84	11.20	104	13.87
5	0.67	25	3.33	45	6.00	65	8.67	85	11.33	105	14.00
6	0.80	26	3.47	46	6.13	66	8.80	86	11.47	106	14.13
7	0.93	27	3.60	47	6.27	67	8.93	87	11.60	107	14.27
8	1.07	28	3.73	48	6.40	68	9.07	88	11.73	108	14.40
9	1.20	29	3.87	49	6.53	69	9.20	89	11.87	109	14.53
10	1.33	30	4.00	50	6.67	70	9.33	90	12.00	110	14.67
11	1.47	31	4.13	51	6.80	71	9.47	91	12.13	111	14.80
12	1.60	32	4.27	52	6.93	72	9.60	92	12.27	112	14.93
13	1.73	33	4.40	53	7.07	73	9.73	93	12.40	113	15.07
14	1.87	34	4.53	54	7.20	74	9.87	94	12.53	114	15.20
15	2.00	35	4.67	55	7.33	75	10.00	95	12.67	115	15.33
16	2.13	36	4.80	56	7.47	76	10.13	96	12.80	116	15.47
17	2.27	37	4.93	57	7.60	77	10.27	97	12.93	117	15.60
18	2.40	38	5.07	58	7.73	78	10.40	98	13.07	118	15.73
19	2.53	39	5.20	59	7.87	79	10.53	99	13.20	119	15.87
20	2.67	40	5.33	60	8.00	80	10.67	100	13.33	120	16.00

Magnesium Sulfate

Pharmacology

Metabolic cofactor involved in both Na-K^+-ATPase and calcium ATPase pumps

Anticonvulsant effects achieved by CNS depression and blockade of peripheral neuromuscular transmission—mechanism believed to be reduced acetylcholine release at motor end plate

Decreases systemic vascular resistance and blood pressure

May depress sinus node and atrioventricular node conduction and myocardial contractility

1 g of magnesium sulfate furnishes 8.12 mEq of magnesium

Administrative Guidelines

Administer infusion via precision control device

Carefully monitor serum levels, electrolytes, ECG, and vital signs

When repeated or continuous doses given, monitor knee jerk reflexes and do not give if patellar reflexes are absent—may cause respiratory depression

Dilute IV infusion solutions to a concentration of less than 20% before administration

Do not administer if spontaneous respiratory rate less than 16 per minute or urine output less than 100 mL for previous 4 hours

Do not admix with alcohol, alkaline solutions, arsenates, barium, calcium, heavy metals, clindamycin, hydrocortisone, polymyxin, tartrates, salicylates, procaine, phosphates, and strontium

Rapid administration may precipitate life-threatening dysrhythmias, cardiac arrest, and respiratory depression

(continued below)

Indications

Prevention and management of seizures in preeclampsia and eclampsia

Control of seizures in hypothyroidism, glomerulonephritis, and epilepsy

Treatment of acute magnesium deficiency and prophylaxis against hypomagnesemia associated with parenteral nutrition

Treatment of acute barium poisoning

Unlabeled Uses. Management of uterine tetany, acute asthma (bronchodilator), cerebral edema (osmotic effects), refractory paroxysmal atrial tachycardia, torsades de pointes, life-threatening ventricular dysrhythmias, acute myocardial infarction, and tetany

Pharmacokinetics

Onset of Action. Immediate

Peak Effects. Within 30 minutes

Duration of Action. About 30 minutes

Metabolism. Excreted by the kidneys proportional to serum concentration

Levels greater than 10 mEq/L may be life-threatening

IV calcium should be readily available to manage overdosage

Contraindicated in acute myocardial damage, heart block, or 2 hours before delivery in toxemia of pregnancy

Use with caution in patients with renal impairment and severe bradydysrhythmias and the elderly. Severe cases may require artificial ventilation, temporary pacemaker insertion, and dialysis

Overdosage may manifest as hypotension, respiratory paralysis, heart block, confusion, and hyporeflexia. Manage with supportive measures and consider 10–20 mL of 10% calcium gluconate or chloride intravenously. Physostigmine 0.5–1.0 mg subcutaneously may be helpful

Magnesium Sulfate

Dosing Information

Preeclampsia and Eclampsia. Initial dose of 4 g (32 mEq) by IV infusion at 150 mg/min. Concomitantly administer 4–5 g (32–40 mEq) IM into each buttock

Subsequent Dosing. 4–5 g (32–40 mEq) undiluted 50% injection IM into alternate buttocks at 4-hour intervals or 1–2 g (8–16 mEq) IV infusion

Total Parenteral Nutrition. 0.5–3.0 g (4–24 mEq) IV daily

Acute Barium Poisoning. 1–2 g (8–16 mEq) IV

Seizures Associated with Epilepsy, Nephritis, and Hypothyroidism. 1 g (8 mEq) IV

Ventricular Dysrhythmias. Initial dose of 2–6 g (6–48 mEq) IV over several minutes

Subsequent Dosing. 3–20 mg/min for up to 48 hours

Acute Myocadial Infarction. 22 g (176 mEq) in 1 L 5% dextrose injection USP at 90 mL/hour over 3 hours. Then 22 mL/hour over the next 21 hours, then 11 mL/hour over the next 24 hours

(continued below)

Potential Drug Interactions

Antagonism of Magnesium Sulfate Effects. Calcium

Possibly Potentiated by Magnesium Sulfate. Digitalis, barbiturates, opiates, general anesthetics, CNS depressants, and neuromuscular blocking agents such as succinylcholine

Principal Adverse Effects

Pulmonary. Respiratory depression

CNS. Loss of reflexes, flaccid paralysis, tetany

CV. Hypotension, cardiac arrest, heart block, bradydysrhythmias, ventricular dysrhythmias

Miscellaneous. Hypocalcemia, flushing, hypothermia, diaphoresis

Paroxysmal Atrial Tachycardia. 3–4 g (24–32 mEq) over 30 seconds with ***extreme caution***

Infusion Rate for Emergency Situations. 2 g (16 mEq) over 1 min, then 5 g over 6 hours

Infusion Rate for Urgent Situations. 1–2 g (8–16 mEq) over 5–60 minutes, then 0.5–1 g (4–8 mEq) per hour for up to 24 hours

Infusion Rate for Nonurgent situations. 50–125 mg/kg over 24 hours

Maximum Infusion Concentration. 200 mg/mL (20%)

Average Infusion Rate. 50 mg/min

Maximum Infusion Rate. 150 mg/min in general situations. Do not exceed 1.2 mEq/min of 10% concentration (or equivalent) except in seizures associated with severe eclampsia

Normal Serum Magnesium Levels. 1.5–2.5 mEq/L

Magnesium Sulfate

How Supplied

10% injection (0.1 g, 0.8 mEq/mL)—
10-mL ampuls of 8 mEq
20-mL ampuls and vials of 16 mEq

12.5% injection (0.125 g, 1.0 mEq/mL)—
8-mL vials of 8 mEq

25% injection (0.25 g, 2.0 mEq/mL)—
vials of 5 mL (10 mEq), 10 mL (20 mEq), 30 mL (60 mEq), 50 mL (100 mEq), and 150 mL (300 mEq)
disposable syringes of 5 mL (10 mEq) and 10 mL (20 mEq)

50% injection (0.50 g, 4.0 mEq/mL)—
2-mL ampuls of 8 mEq
10-mL ampuls of 40 mEq

Magnesium Sulfate

22 g in 500 mL

■ Infusion Rate in mL/hr (pump setting) ■ Drug Dose in g/hr

mL/hr	g/hr	mL/hr	g/hr	mL/hr	g/hr	mL/hr	g/hr	mL/hr	g/hr	mL/hr	g/hr
1	0.04	21	0.92	41	1.80	61	2.68	81	3.56	101	4.44
2	0.08	22	0.96	42	1.84	62	2.72	82	3.60	102	4.48
3	0.13	23	1.01	43	1.89	63	2.77	83	3.65	103	4.53
4	0.17	24	1.05	44	1.93	64	2.81	84	3.69	104	4.57
5	0.22	25	1.10	45	1.98	65	2.86	85	3.74	105	4.62
6	0.26	26	1.14	46	2.02	66	2.90	86	3.78	106	4.66
7	0.30	27	1.18	47	2.06	67	2.94	87	3.82	107	4.70
8	0.35	28	1.23	48	2.11	68	2.99	88	3.87	108	4.75
9	0.39	29	1.27	49	2.15	69	3.03	89	3.91	109	4.79
10	0.44	30	1.32	50	2.20	70	3.08	90	3.96	110	4.84
11	0.48	31	1.36	51	2.24	71	3.12	91	4.00	111	4.88
12	0.52	32	1.40	52	2.28	72	3.16	92	4.04	112	4.92
13	0.57	33	1.45	53	2.33	73	3.21	93	4.09	113	4.97
14	0.61	34	1.49	54	2.37	74	3.25	94	4.13	114	5.01
15	0.66	35	1.54	55	2.42	75	3.30	95	4.18	115	5.06
16	0.70	36	1.58	56	2.46	76	3.34	96	4.22	116	5.10
17	0.74	37	1.62	57	2.50	77	3.38	97	4.26	117	5.14
18	0.79	38	1.67	58	2.55	78	3.43	98	4.31	118	5.19
19	0.83	39	1.71	59	2.59	79	3.47	99	4.35	119	5.23
20	0.88	40	1.76	60	2.64	80	3.52	100	4.40	120	5.28

■ Infusion Rate in mL/hr (pump setting) ■ **Drug Dose in g/hr**

mL/hr	g/hr	mL/hr	g/hr	mL/hr	g/hr	mL/hr	g/hr	mL/hr	g/hr	mL/hr	g/hr
1	0.02	21	0.46	41	0.90	61	1.34	81	1.78	101	2.22
2	0.04	22	0.48	42	0.92	62	1.36	82	1.80	102	2.24
3	0.06	23	0.50	43	0.94	63	1.38	83	1.82	103	2.26
4	0.08	24	0.52	44	0.96	64	1.40	84	1.84	104	2.28
5	0.11	25	0.55	45	0.99	65	1.43	85	1.87	105	2.31
6	0.13	26	0.57	46	1.01	66	1.45	86	1.89	106	2.33
7	0.15	27	0.59	47	1.03	67	1.47	87	1.91	107	2.35
8	0.17	28	0.61	48	1.05	68	1.49	88	1.93	108	2.37
9	0.19	29	0.63	49	1.07	69	1.51	89	1.95	109	2.39
10	0.22	30	0.66	50	1.10	70	1.54	90	1.98	110	2.42
11	0.24	31	0.68	51	1.12	71	1.56	91	2.00	111	2.44
12	0.26	32	0.70	52	1.14	72	1.58	92	2.02	112	2.46
13	0.28	33	0.72	53	1.16	73	1.60	93	2.04	113	2.48
14	0.30	34	0.74	54	1.18	74	1.62	94	2.06	114	2.50
15	0.33	35	0.77	55	1.21	75	1.65	95	2.09	115	2.53
16	0.35	36	0.79	56	1.23	76	1.67	96	2.11	116	2.55
17	0.37	37	0.81	57	1.25	77	1.69	97	2.13	117	2.57
18	0.39	38	0.83	58	1.27	78	1.71	98	2.15	118	2.59
19	0.41	39	0.85	59	1.29	79	1.73	99	2.17	119	2.61
20	0.44	40	0.88	60	1.32	80	1.76	100	2.20	120	2.64

Mannitol (Osmitrol)

Pharmacology

Osmotic diuretic that inhibits tubular reabsorption of water and solutes

May increase renal blood flow and protect the kidney against nephrotoxin accumulation in tubular fluid following trauma. This may prevent or reverse acute renal failure

Promotes fluid shift from erythrocytes to plasma and cells to extracellular fluid, thereby diminishing cerebral edema by reducing cerebrospinal fluid pressure and brain mass

Increases extracellular volume, plasma volume, and circulation time but decreases hematocrit, serum sodium, and pH

Reduces intraocular pressure by fluid egress from the anterior chamber of the eye

Administrative Guidelines

Administer infusion via precision control device

Monitor urine output, renal function, CBC, electrolytes, and central venous pressure and watch for signs of heart failure

Employ filter in infusion line and do not administer with blood

Solutions greater than 15% have a tendency to crystallize at low temperatures. Warm to dissolve crystals, let cool to body temperature before infusing, and discard if crystals cannot be removed

Correct electrolytes, acid-base status, hemoglobin, and plasma volume before use

Decrease or discontinue infusion if no clinical response noted, urine output falls, or heart failure occurs

Avoid extravasation because skin necrosis may ensue

Contraindicated in patients with renal impairment who do not respond to a test dose; severe heart disease; pulmonary edema; severe dehydration; documented

(continued below)

Indications

Promotes diuresis in the prevention and treatment of the oliguric phase of acute renal failure. No appreciable effect once tubular necrosis has occurred

Prevents hemoglobin buildup during cardiopulmonary bypass

Prophylaxis against renal tubular insults in high-risk patients undergoing surgical procedures

Reduction of intracranial pressure before and during neurosurgery and in patients with diabetic ketoacidosis or hypoglycemic coma

Lowers intraocular pressure; promotes urinary excretion of toxins in drug poisonings; enhances uric acid excretion; and is used as treatment of ethylene glycol and carbon monoxide poisoning

acute tubular necrosis; active intracranial bleeding unrelated to craniotomy; and metabolic edema associated with increased capillary permeability unrelated to renal, hepatic, or cardiac disorders

Use with caution in patients with shock and uncertain renal status

Overdosage requires discontinuation of infusion, supportive measures, and correction of fluid and electrolyte imbalance. Hemodialysis may be beneficial

Mannitol (Osmitrol)

Pharmacokinetics

Onset of Action. 15–60 minutes

Peak Effects. 60 minutes

Duration of Action. 6–8 hours

Elimination Half-Life. Approximately 100 minutes

Metabolism. Minimally via liver to glycogen with renal elimination by glomerular filtration

Dosing Information

Test Dose in Marked Oliguria or Suspected Tubular Damage. 0.2 g/kg or 12.5 g over 3–5 minutes. May repeat after 2–3 hours if urine output is less than 30–50 mL/hour

Prevention of Oliguric Renal Failure. 50–100 g over 90 minutes to several hours

Reduction of Intracranial/Intraocular Pressure. 1.5–2.0 g/kg over 30–60 minutes

Drug Intoxications. 0.5 g/kg or 25–50 g initially over 5–10 minutes, then 5–10% solution at a rate to maintain urine output at 100–500 mL/hour

Maximum Dose. Rarely greater than 200 g over 24 hours

How Supplied

5% solution in 1000 mL (275 mOsm/L)

10% solution in 500 mL and 1000 mL (550 mOsm/L)

15% solution in 150 mL and 500 mL (825 mOsm/L)

20% solution in 250 mL and 500 mL (1100 mOsm/L)

25% solution in 50 mL (1375 mOsm/L)

Potential Drug Interactions

Possibly Antagonized by Mannitol. Lithium

Principal Adverse Effects

CNS. Headaches, disorientation, nausea, vomiting, syncope, coma, muscle rigidity, death

CV. Tachycardia, hypotension, heart failure, hypertension, chest pain

Renal. Acidosis, oliguric renal failure, urinary retention, uricosuria

Miscellaneous. Fever; chills; rhinitis; backache; infusion site phlebitis and skin necrosis; urticaria; alteration of electrolyte, phosphorus, and ethylene glycol measurements

Mannitol (Osmitrol) — 100 g in 500 mL

■ **Infusion Rate in mL/hr (pump setting)** ■ **Drug Dose in g/hr**

mL/hr	g/hr	mL/hr	g/hr	mL/hr	g/hr	mL/hr	g/hr	mL/hr	g/hr	mL/hr	g/hr
1	0.20	21	4.20	41	8.20	61	12.20	81	16.20	101	20.20
2	0.40	22	4.40	42	8.40	62	12.40	82	16.40	102	20.40
3	0.60	23	4.60	43	8.60	63	12.60	83	16.60	103	20.60
4	0.80	24	4.80	44	8.80	64	12.80	84	16.80	104	20.80
5	1.00	25	5.00	45	9.00	65	13.00	85	17.00	105	21.00
6	1.20	26	5.20	46	9.20	66	13.20	86	17.20	106	21.20
7	1.40	27	5.40	47	9.40	67	13.40	87	17.40	107	21.40
8	1.60	28	5.60	48	9.60	68	13.60	88	17.60	108	21.60
9	1.80	29	5.80	49	9.80	69	13.80	89	17.80	109	21.80
10	2.00	30	6.00	50	10.00	70	14.00	90	18.00	110	22.00
11	2.20	31	6.20	51	10.20	71	14.20	91	18.20	111	22.20
12	2.40	32	6.40	52	10.40	72	14.40	92	18.40	112	22.40
13	2.60	33	6.60	53	10.60	73	14.60	93	18.60	113	22.60
14	2.80	34	6.80	54	10.80	74	14.80	94	18.80	114	22.80
15	3.00	35	7.00	55	11.00	75	15.00	95	19.00	115	23.00
16	3.20	36	7.20	56	11.20	76	15.20	96	19.20	116	23.20
17	3.40	37	7.40	57	11.40	77	15.40	97	19.40	117	23.40
18	3.60	38	7.60	58	11.60	78	15.60	98	19.60	118	23.60
19	3.80	39	7.80	59	11.80	79	15.80	99	19.80	119	23.80
20	4.00	40	4.00	60	12.00	80	16.00	100	20.00	120	24.00

Infusion Rate in mL/hr (pump setting)	Drug Dose in g/hr	Infusion Rate in mL/hr (pump setting)	Drug Dose in g/hr	Infusion Rate in mL/hr (pump setting)	Drug Dose in g/hr	Infusion Rate in mL/hr (pump setting)	Drug Dose in g/hr	Infusion Rate in mL/hr (pump setting)	Drug Dose in g/hr	Infusion Rate in mL/hr (pump setting)	Drug Dose in g/hr
1	0.10	21	2.10	41	4.10	61	6.10	81	8.10	101	10.10
2	0.20	22	2.20	42	4.20	62	6.20	82	8.20	102	10.20
3	0.30	23	2.30	43	4.30	63	6.30	83	8.30	103	10.30
4	0.40	24	2.40	44	4.40	64	6.40	84	8.40	104	10.40
5	0.50	25	2.50	45	4.50	65	6.50	85	8.50	105	10.50
6	0.60	26	2.60	46	4.60	66	6.60	86	8.60	106	10.60
7	0.70	27	2.70	47	4.70	67	6.70	87	8.70	107	10.70
8	0.80	28	2.80	48	4.80	68	6.80	88	8.80	108	10.80
9	0.90	29	2.90	49	4.90	69	6.90	89	8.90	109	10.90
10	1.00	30	3.00	50	5.00	70	7.00	90	9.00	110	11.00
11	1.10	31	3.10	51	5.10	71	7.10	91	9.10	111	11.10
12	1.20	32	3.20	52	5.20	72	7.20	92	9.20	112	11.20
13	1.30	33	3.30	53	5.30	73	7.30	93	9.30	113	11.30
14	1.40	34	3.40	54	5.40	74	7.40	94	9.40	114	11.40
15	1.50	35	3.50	55	5.50	75	7.50	95	9.50	115	11.50
16	1.60	36	3.60	56	5.60	76	7.60	96	9.60	116	11.60
17	1.70	37	3.70	57	5.70	77	7.70	97	9.70	117	11.70
18	1.80	38	3.80	58	5.80	78	7.80	98	9.80	118	11.80
19	1.90	39	3.90	59	5.90	79	7.90	99	9.90	119	11.90
20	2.00	40	4.00	60	6.00	80	8.00	100	10.00	120	12.00

Metoprolol (Lopressor)

Pharmacology

Competitive $beta_1$ selective adrenoreceptor blocking agent

Principal effects exerted on myocardial $beta_1$ receptors; affects $beta_2$ receptors in bronchial and vascular smooth muscle only at high doses

Reduces myocardial contractility, resting heart rate, blood pressure, reflex orthostatic tachycardia, and cardiac output at rest and during exercise without compensatory rise in total peripheral resistance

Decreases myocardial automaticity and conduction velocity through the sinoatrial and atrioventricular nodes

Increases cardiac volume and systolic ejection time, but does not alter stroke volume

Beneficial response in patients with angina is likely mediated by blockade of catecholamine effects, thereby reducing myocardial oxygen consumption

(continued below)

Administrative Guidelines

Carefully monitor ECG, vital signs, and, if available, hemodynamic variables

Administer as soon as feasible to patients with acute myocardial infarction

Avoid abrupt cessation of ***long-term*** therapy in patients with ischemic heart disease—may precipitate angina or acute myocardial infarction. Suggest low dose or tapering therapy over 1–2 weeks to avoid catecholamine rebound responses

Contraindicated in those with known hypersensitivity, second-degree or third-degree heart block, sinus bradycardia, cardiogenic shock, severe heart failure unrelated to tachydysrhythmias requiring beta-blockers, and acute myocardial infarction associated with heart rate <45 bpm, P-R interval ≥ 0.24 second; moderate-to-severe heart failure; and a systolic blood pressure <100 mmHg

(continued below)

Reduces incidence of ventricular fibrillation, risk of reinfarction, and long-term mortality in patients with acute myocardial infarction—may reduce infarct size if employed early

May block renin and insulin release, raise serum potassium and triglyceride levels, blunt increases in exercise-induced plasma glycerol, and elevate peripheral platelet counts

No significant intrinsic sympathomimetic or membrane stabilizing activity

Moderately lipophilic

Indications

Management of hemodynamically stable patients with suspected or proven acute myocardial infarction

Treatment of chronic stable angina pectoris

Control of essential hypertension

Unlabeled Uses. Management of multifocal atrial tachycardia

Use with extreme caution in patients with bronchospastic disease and concomitantly administer a $beta_2$ agonist

Use with caution in those with diabetes, suspected thyrotoxicosis, heart failure, cardiomegaly; during general anesthesia for major surgery; in those with peripheral vascular disease, impaired hepatic function, pheochromocytoma, and sinoatrial or atrioventricular node dysfunction

Overdosage may manifest with bradycardia, heart block, hypotension, heart failure, bronchospasm, shock, altered mental status with seizures or coma, and hyperkalemia or hypoglycemia. Manage with general supportive measures, and consider atropine, glucagon, isoproterenol, epinephrine, and pacing for bradydysrhythmias; theophylline and $beta_2$ agonists for bronchospasm; vasopressors for hypotension; and inotropic therapy for cardiac failure. There is no established role for dialysis

Metoprolol (Lopressor)

Pharmacokinetics

Onset of Action. Within 20 minutes

Peak Effects. Approximately 20 minutes

Duration of Action. Approximately 5 hours after 5-mg IV dose and 8 hours after 15-mg IV dose

Elimination Half-Life. 3–7 hours

Metabolism. Via hydroxylation in liver with renal elimination of primarily inactive metabolites

Dosing Information

Myocardial Infarction. Three 5-mg IV doses by rapid injection at approximately 2-minute intervals. Begin oral therapy after 15 minutes ***only*** if hemodynamically stable with 50 mg orally every 6 hours for 48 hours, then 100 mg twice daily. If initial IV bolus dosing is not tolerated, begin oral therapy when hemodynamically stable or 15 minutes after the last IV dose. Administer 25–50 mg orally every 6 hours for 48 hours, then 100 mg orally twice daily

How Supplied

1 mg/mL—5-mL ampuls of 5 mg

Potential Drug Interactions

Potentiation of Metoprolol Effects. Antihypertensive drugs, diuretics, verapamil, catecholamine-depleting agents such as reserpine, cardiac glycosides, myocardial depressants, general anesthetics such as dimethyl ether, oral contraceptives, flecainide, haloperidol, hydralazine, monoamine oxidase inhibitors, cimetidine, ranitidine, propafenone, quinidine, calcium channel blockers, quinolones, thioamines, phenytoin, lidocaine, procainamide, disopyramide

Antagonism of Metoprolol Effects. Thyroid hormones, $beta_1$ and $beta_2$ agonists

Possibly Potentiated by Metoprolol. Prazosin, cardiac glycosides, lidocaine, ergot alkaloids, clonidine, epinephrine, hydralazine, flecainide, benzodiazepines, warfarin

Possibly Antagonized by Metoprolol. Sulfonylureas

Metoprolol (Lopressor)

Principal Adverse Effects

CNS. Weakness, altered mental status, insomnia, nightmares, hallucinations, somnolence, dizziness, headache, nervousness, visual disturbances, depression, catatonia, impotence, lethargy, emotional lability, and short-term memory loss

Pulmonary. Dyspnea and bronchospasm with wheezing

CV. Bradycardia, hypotension, heart failure, heart block, cardiac arrest, palpitations, chest pain, peripheral edema and arterial insufficiency, Raynaud's phenomenon, syncope, and pericarditis

GI. Nausea, abdominal pain, diarrhea, flatulence, constipation, xerostomia, hiccups, heartburn, and elevated liver function tests

Renal. Decreased renal blood flow; elevations of blood urea nitrogen, creatinine, and uric acid

Heme. Agranulocytosis, eosinophilia, and thrombocytopenic and nonthrombocytopenic purpura

(continued below)

Dermatological. Maculopapular rash, urticaria, pruritus, dry skin, worsening of psoriasis, and alopecia

Miscellaneous. Variable antinuclear factor levels, decreased libido, diaphoresis, blurred vision, dry eyes and mucous membranes, Peyronie's disease, polymyalgia-like syndrome, and tinnitus

Midazolam Hydrochloride (Versed)

Pharmacology

Short-acting benzodiazepine with dose-dependent CNS depressant effects at the hypothalamic, thalamic, and limbic levels

Mechanism of action may be neurotransmitter inhibition of gamma-aminobutyric acid

Diminishes anxiety and promotes sedation, hypnosis, antegrade amnesia, and skeletal muscle relaxation

May decrease intraocular pressure, mean arterial blood pressure, cardiac output, stroke volume, and peripheral vascular resistance

Respiratory mechanics are not impaired, but ventilatory response to carbon dioxide stimulation may be blunted

Decreases cerebrospinal fluid pressure in the absence of intracranial lesions. Conversely, may augment cerebrospinal fluid pressure when intracranial pathology is present

Highly protein bound—three to four times more potent than diazepam

Administrative Guidelines

Administer infusion via precision control device

Continuously monitor ECG and vital signs during administration and recovery

Always ensure that oxygen, resuscitative equipment, and trained personnel are immediately available

Do not administer rapidly or by single IV bolus dose for conscious sedation

Avoid intra-arterial administration

Employ reduced dose in elderly patients and anticipate either a profound or prolonged response

Observe patients for 3–6 hours following intravenous use, and caution against operating hazardous machinery, driving, or partaking in activities requiring complete mental alertness

Midazolam has abuse potential and may cause physical dependence

(continued below)

Indications

Induction of sedation, light anesthesia, and amnesia before endoscopic procedures, cardiac catheterization, and other short diagnostic studies

Adjunct to induction of general anesthesia and maintenance of anesthesia during short surgical procedures

Unlabeled Uses. Before dental procedures or DC cardioversion; acute agitation disorders; anticonvulsant for seizure control

Pharmacokinetics

Onset of Action. 1–5 minutes after IV bolus

Peak Effects. Within 1 hour

Duration of Action. 2–6 hours

Plasma (Distribution) Half-Life. 6–20 minutes

Tissue (Elimination) Half-Life. 1.2–12.3 hours

Metabolism. Via hydroxylation in liver with excretion of conjugated metabolites by the kidney

Contraindicated with known hypersensitivity, narrow-angle glaucoma, untreated open-angle glaucoma, shock, coma, and acute alcohol intoxication with depressed vital signs

Use with caution in older or debilitated patients; those with decreased pulmonary reserve, renal insufficiency, congestive heart failure; individuals performing hazardous tasks or skills requiring mental acuity; high-risk surgical patients; uncompensated acute illnesses especially in association with fluid and electrolyte disturbances, and with narcotics, barbiturates, alcohol, or other CNS depressants

Overdosage may manifest as somnolence, confusion, diminished reflexes, altered vital signs, and coma. Manage with general supportive measures and careful monitoring. Flumazenil should also be used to reverse partial or complete sedation and other pharmacologic effects. There is no established role for dialysis

Midazolam Hydrochloride (Versed)

Dosing Information

Conscious Sedation for Endoscopic or Cardiovascular Procedures

Unpremedicated Healthy Adults Under 60 Years Old. 1–2.5 mg IV over at least 2–3 minutes. Wait at least 2 minutes to assess clinical response and repeat dose if necessary

Premedicated Healthy Adults Under 60 Years Old. 70% of "unpremedicated adults under 60" dose (0.7–1.8 mg) usually required

Maximum Dose Recommended. 0.1–0.15 mg/kg but rarely greater than 5 mg total dose is indicated

Unpremedicated Adults Over 60 Years Old, Chronically Ill or Debilitated Patients, and Those with Decreased Pulmonary Reserve. 1–1.5 mg IV over at least 2–3 minutes. May repeat after at least 2 minutes observation using incremental doses of 1 mg or less

(continued below)

Potential Drug Interactions

Potentiation of Midazolam Effects. Narcotics, barbiturates, alcohol, cardiorespiratory depressants, cimetidine, droperidol

Antagonism of Midazolam Effects. Theophylline

Possibly Potentiated by Midazolam. Thiopental, halothane, alcohol, barbiturates, CNS depressants, sedatives, other anesthetics, narcotics, and analgesics

Possibly Antagonized by Midazolam. Ketamine

Premedicated Adults Over 60 Years Old, Chronically Ill or Debilitated Patients, and Those with Decreased Pulmonary Reserve. 50% of "unpremedicated adults over 60" dose (0.5–0.75 mg) is usually required

Maximum Dose Recommended. Rarely greater than 3.5 mg total dose is indicated

Maintenance Dose for Conscious Sedation. Administer 25% incremental doses of the total dose first required to achieve a sedative state

(continued on page 174)

Principal Adverse Effects

CNS. Headache, altered states of consciousness, somnolence, coma, paresthesias, insomnia, anxiety, retrograde amnesia, ataxia, increased cough reflex, dysphonia, athetoid movements, sleep disturbances, dizziness, prolonged anesthesia recovery, nystagmus, diplopia, lightheadedness, visual and auditory disturbances, pinpoint pupils, yawning, and hyporeflexia

Pulmonary. Apnea, respiratory arrest, laryngospasm, bronchospasm, tachypnea, dyspnea, hyperventilation

CV. Hypotension, vasovagal responses, ventricular extrasystole, tachycardia, junctional rhythm, bradycardia

GI. Nausea, vomiting, excessive salivation, acid taste

Dermatological. Phlebitis, warmth, coldness at injection site, rash, urticaria, pruritus

Miscellaneous. Chills, hiccups, weakness, toothache, hematoma

Midazolam Hydrochloride (Versed)

Induction of Anesthesia—Before Other Anesthetics

Unpremedicated Adults Under 55 Years Old. 0.2–0.35 mg/kg IV bolus over 20–30 seconds initially. After 2 minutes observation, may repeat with 25% of initial dose (0.05–0.10 mg/kg) as necessary

Maximum Dose Recommended. 0.6 mg/kg

Premedicated Adults Under 55 Years Old. 0.25 mg/kg IV bolus over 20–30 seconds initially. After 2 minutes observation, may repeat with 25% of initial dose (0.06 mg/kg) as necessary

Unpremedicated Adults Over 55 Years Old. 0.3 mg/kg IV bolus over 20–30 seconds. After 2 minutes observation, may repeat with 25% of initial dose (0.08 mg/kg) as necessary

Unpremedicated Adults Over 55 Years Old with Severe or Debilitating Illness. 0.15–0.25 mg/kg IV bolus over 20–30 seconds initially. After 2 minutes observation, may repeat with 25% of initial dose (0.04–0.06 mg/kg) as necessary

(continued below)

Premedicated Healthy Adults Over 55 Years Old. 0.2 mg/kg IV bolus over 20–30 seconds initially. After 2 minutes observation, may repeat with 25% of initial dose (0.05 mg/kg) as necessary

Premedicated Adults Over 55 Years Old with Severe or Debilitating Illness. 0.15 mg/kg IV bolus over 20–30 seconds initially. After 2 minutes observation, may repeat with 25% of initial dose (0.04 mg/kg) as necessary

Maintenance Dose for Anesthesia. Administer 25% incremental doses of the total dose first required to achieve induction

How Supplied

1 mg/mL—2-mL vials of 2 mg
5-mL vials of 5 mg
10-mL vials of 10 mg

5 mg/mL—1-mL vials of 5 mg
2-mL vials and syringes of 10 mg
5-mL vials of 25 mg
10-mL vials of 50 mg

Midazolam Hydrochloride (Versed) 100 mg in 250 mL

■ **Infusion Rate in mL/hr (pump setting)** ■ **Drug Dose in mg/hr**

mL/hr	mg/hr	mL/hr	mg/hr	mL/hr	mg/hr	mL/hr	mg/hr	mL/hr	mg/hr	mL/hr	mg/hr
1	0.4	21	8.4	41	16.4	61	24.4	81	32.4	101	40.4
2	0.8	22	8.8	42	16.8	62	24.8	82	32.8	102	40.8
3	1.2	23	9.2	43	17.2	63	25.2	83	33.2	103	41.2
4	1.6	24	9.6	44	17.6	64	25.6	84	33.6	104	41.6
5	2.0	25	10.0	45	18.0	65	26.0	85	34.0	105	42.0
6	2.4	26	10.4	46	18.4	66	26.4	86	34.4	106	42.4
7	2.8	27	10.8	47	18.8	67	26.8	87	34.8	107	42.8
8	3.2	28	11.2	48	19.2	68	27.2	88	35.2	108	43.2
9	3.6	29	11.6	49	19.6	69	27.6	89	35.6	109	43.6
10	4.0	30	12.0	50	20.0	70	28.0	90	36.0	110	44.0
11	4.4	31	12.4	51	20.4	71	28.4	91	36.4	111	44.4
12	4.8	32	12.8	52	20.8	72	28.8	92	36.8	112	44.8
13	5.2	33	13.2	53	21.2	73	29.2	93	37.2	113	45.2
14	5.6	34	13.6	54	21.6	74	29.6	94	37.6	114	45.6
15	6.0	35	14.0	55	22.0	75	30.0	95	38.0	115	46.0
16	6.4	36	14.4	56	22.4	76	30.4	96	38.4	116	46.4
17	6.8	37	14.8	57	22.8	77	30.8	97	38.8	117	46.8
18	7.2	38	15.2	58	23.2	78	31.2	98	39.2	118	47.2
19	7.6	39	15.6	59	23.6	79	31.6	99	39.6	119	47.6
20	8.0	40	16.0	60	24.0	80	32.0	100	40.0	120	48.0

DRUG DOSE in mg/kg/hr

Patient's Weight; rows: Infusion Rate in mL/hr

kg / lbs	40 / 88	45 / 99	50 / 110	55 / 121	60 / 132	65 / 143	70 / 154	75 / 165	80 / 176	85 / 187	90 / 198	95 / 209	100 / 220	105 / 231	110 / 242
5	0.05	0.04	0.04	0.04	0.03	0.03	0.03	0.03	0.03	0.02	0.02	0.02	0.02	0.02	0.02
10	0.10	0.09	0.08	0.07	0.07	0.06	0.06	0.05	0.05	0.05	0.04	0.04	0.04	0.04	0.04
15	0.15	0.13	0.12	0.11	0.10	0.09	0.09	0.08	0.08	0.07	0.07	0.06	0.06	0.06	0.05
20	0.20	0.18	0.16	0.15	0.13	0.12	0.11	0.11	0.10	0.09	0.09	0.08	0.08	0.08	0.07
25	0.25	0.22	0.20	0.18	0.17	0.15	0.14	0.13	0.13	0.12	0.11	0.11	0.10	0.10	0.09
30	0.30	0.27	0.24	0.22	0.20	0.18	0.17	0.16	0.15	0.14	0.13	0.13	0.12	0.11	0.11
35	0.35	0.31	0.28	0.25	0.23	0.22	0.20	0.19	0.17	0.16	0.16	0.15	0.14	0.13	0.13
40	0.40	0.36	0.32	0.29	0.27	0.25	0.23	0.21	0.20	0.19	0.18	0.17	0.16	0.15	0.15
45	0.45	0.40	0.36	0.33	0.30	0.28	0.26	0.24	0.22	0.21	0.20	0.19	0.18	0.17	0.16
50	0.50	0.44	0.40	0.36	0.33	0.31	0.29	0.27	0.25	0.24	0.22	0.21	0.20	0.19	0.18
55	0.55	0.49	0.44	0.40	0.37	0.34	0.31	0.29	0.28	0.26	0.24	0.23	0.22	0.21	0.20
60	0.60	0.53	0.48	0.44	0.40	0.37	0.34	0.32	0.30	0.28	0.27	0.25	0.24	0.23	0.22
65	0.65	0.58	0.52	0.47	0.43	0.40	0.37	0.35	0.32	0.31	0.29	0.27	0.26	0.25	0.24
70	0.70	0.62	0.56	0.51	0.47	0.43	0.40	0.37	0.35	0.33	0.31	0.29	0.28	0.27	0.25
75	0.75	0.67	0.60	0.55	0.50	0.46	0.43	0.40	0.38	0.35	0.33	0.32	0.30	0.29	0.27
80	0.80	0.71	0.64	0.58	0.53	0.49	0.46	0.43	0.40	0.38	0.36	0.34	0.32	0.30	0.29
85	0.85	0.76	0.68	0.62	0.57	0.52	0.49	0.45	0.43	0.40	0.38	0.36	0.34	0.32	0.31
90	0.90	0.80	0.72	0.65	0.60	0.55	0.51	0.48	0.45	0.42	0.40	0.38	0.36	0.34	0.33
95	0.95	0.84	0.76	0.69	0.63	0.58	0.54	0.51	0.47	0.45	0.42	0.40	0.38	0.36	0.35
100	1.00	0.89	0.80	0.73	0.67	0.62	0.57	0.53	0.50	0.47	0.44	0.42	0.40	0.38	0.36
105	1.05	0.93	0.84	0.76	0.70	0.65	0.60	0.56	0.52	0.49	0.47	0.44	0.42	0.40	0.38
110	1.10	0.98	0.88	0.80	0.73	0.68	0.63	0.59	0.55	0.52	0.49	0.46	0.44	0.42	0.40
115	1.15	1.02	0.92	0.84	0.77	0.71	0.66	0.61	0.57	0.54	0.51	0.48	0.46	0.44	0.42
120	1.20	1.07	0.96	0.87	0.80	0.74	0.69	0.64	0.60	0.56	0.53	0.51	0.48	0.46	0.44

Milrinone Lactate (Primacor)

Pharmacology

Selectively inhibits peak III cyclic adenosine monophosphate phosphodiesterase isozyme in vascular and cardiac muscle, thereby increasing intracellular ionized calcium

Dose-dependent positive inotropic and vasodilator effects with minimal chronotropic response

Decreases pulmonary capillary wedge pressure and peripheral vascular resistance and increases cardiac output

Improves diastolic relaxation and left ventricular function

No significant increase in myocardial oxygen consumption

Indications

Short-term (less than 5 days) management of congestive heart failure

Administrative Guidelines

Administer infusion via precision control device

Continuously monitor ECG, blood pressure, and vital signs

Follow hemodynamics, electrolytes, renal function, and acid-base status

Administer via central line, if possible, or large vein

Do not use solution if discolored or particulate matter is present

Diluents of 5% dextrose injections USP, 0.9% sodium chloride injection USP, or 0.45% sodium chloride injection USP may be used to prepare infusion

Correct any underlying hypovolemia, if possible, before use

Correct hypokalemia before and during infusion, especially in digitalized patients

Do not administer furosemide into milrinone infusion line because precipitate may form

(continued below)

Pharmacokinetics

Onset of Action. Within 5–15 minutes

Peak Effects. Not specified by manufacturer

Elimination Half-Life. Approximately 2.3 hours

Metabolism. Renal failure diminishes drug clearance but precise mechanism of metabolism not specified by manufacturer

Decrease infusion rate with renal failure

May aggravate ventricular dysrhythmias

May accelerate ventricular response in patients with atrial fibrillation or flutter. Consider pretreatment with digitalis in these cases

Safety in patients with acute myocardial infarction and pregnancy has not been established

Contraindicated in patients with severe aortic or pulmonic stenosis, obstructive subaortic stenosis, and those with known hypersensitivity

Use cautiously in those with hypovolemia, renal failure, and in nursing mothers

Overdosage may manifest with hypotension and dysrhythmias. Manage with general supportive measures and decrease or terminate infusion

Milrinone Lactate (Primacor)

Dosing Information

Initial Loading Dose. 50 μg/kg over 10 minutes

Minimal Infusion Rate. 0.375 μg/kg/min

Standard Infusion Rate. 0.50 μg/kg/min

Maximum Infusion Rate. 0.75 μg/kg/min

Maximum Daily Dose. 1.13 mg/kg/day

Titration Guideline

Suggested Regimen. Adjust infusion by 0.125 μg/kg/min every 15–30 minutes as necessary guided by hemodynamic response

How Supplied

1 mg/mL—Carpuject sterile cartridge needles of 5 mL (5 mg)
Single-dose vials of 10 mL (10 mg) or 20 mL (20 mg)

Potential Drug Interactions

None specified by manufacturer

Principal Adverse Effects

CNS. Headache, tremor

CV. Ventricular and supraventricular dysrhythmias, hypotension, angina

Heme. Thrombocytopenia

Miscellaneous. Hypokalemia

Milrinone Lactate (Primacor) 20 mg in 150 mL

DRUG DOSE in μg/kg/min

Infusion Rate in mL/hr — Patient's Weight kg / lbs	40 / 88	45 / 99	50 / 110	55 / 121	60 / 132	65 / 143	70 / 154	75 / 165	80 / 176	85 / 187	90 / 198	95 / 209	100 / 220	105 / 231	110 / 242
5	0.27	0.24	0.22	0.20	0.18	0.17	0.15	0.14	0.13	0.13	0.12	0.11	0.11	0.10	0.10
10	0.55	0.49	0.44	0.40	0.37	0.34	0.31	0.29	0.27	0.26	0.24	0.23	0.22	0.21	0.20
15	0.83	0.74	0.66	0.60	0.55	0.51	0.47	0.44	0.41	0.39	0.37	0.35	0.33	0.31	0.30
20	1.11	0.98	0.88	0.80	0.74	0.68	0.63	0.59	0.55	0.52	0.49	0.46	0.44	0.42	0.40
25	1.38	1.23	1.11	1.01	0.92	0.85	0.79	0.74	0.69	0.65	0.61	0.58	0.55	0.52	0.50
30	1.66	1.48	1.33	1.21	1.11	1.02	0.95	0.88	0.83	0.78	0.74	0.70	0.66	0.63	0.60
35	1.94	1.72	1.55	1.41	1.29	1.19	1.11	1.03	0.97	0.91	0.86	0.81	0.77	0.74	0.70
40	2.22	1.97	1.77	1.61	1.48	1.36	1.27	1.18	1.11	1.04	0.98	0.93	0.88	0.84	0.80
45	2.50	2.22	2.00	1.81	1.66	1.53	1.42	1.33	1.25	1.17	1.11	1.05	1.00	0.95	0.90
50	2.77	2.46	2.22	2.02	1.85	1.70	1.58	1.48	1.38	1.30	1.23	1.17	1.11	1.05	1.01
55	3.05	2.71	2.44	2.22	2.03	1.88	1.74	1.63	1.52	1.43	1.35	1.28	1.22	1.16	1.11
60	3.33	2.96	2.66	2.42	2.22	2.05	1.90	1.77	1.66	1.56	1.48	1.40	1.33	1.27	1.21
65	3.61	3.21	2.88	2.62	2.40	2.22	2.06	1.92	1.80	1.69	1.60	1.52	1.44	1.37	1.31
70	3.88	3.45	3.11	2.82	2.59	2.39	2.22	2.07	1.94	1.83	1.72	1.63	1.55	1.48	1.41
75	4.16	3.70	3.33	3.03	2.77	2.56	2.38	2.22	2.08	1.96	1.85	1.75	1.66	1.58	1.51
80	4.44	3.95	3.55	3.23	2.96	2.73	2.54	2.37	2.22	2.09	1.97	1.87	1.77	1.69	1.61
85	4.72	4.19	3.77	3.43	3.14	2.90	2.69	2.51	2.36	2.22	2.09	1.98	1.88	1.79	1.71
90	5.00	4.44	4.00	3.63	3.33	3.07	2.85	2.66	2.50	2.35	2.22	2.10	2.00	1.90	1.81
95	5.27	4.69	4.22	3.83	3.51	3.24	3.01	2.81	2.63	2.48	2.34	2.22	2.11	2.01	1.91
100	5.55	4.93	4.44	4.04	3.70	3.41	3.17	2.96	2.77	1.61	2.46	2.33	2.22	2.11	2.02
105	5.83	5.18	4.66	4.24	3.88	3.59	3.33	3.11	2.91	2.74	2.59	2.45	2.33	2.22	2.12
110	6.11	5.43	4.88	4.44	4.07	3.76	3.49	3.25	3.05	2.87	2.71	2.57	2.44	2.32	2.22
115	6.38	5.67	5.11	4.64	4.25	3.93	3.65	3.40	3.19	3.00	2.84	2.69	2.55	2.43	2.32
120	6.66	5.92	5.33	4.84	4.44	4.10	3.81	3.55	3.33	3.13	2.96	2.80	2.66	2.54	[illegible]

DRUG DOSE in µg/kg/min

Infusion Rate in mL/hr	Patient's Weight kg: 40 (lbs 88)	45 (99)	50 (110)	55 (121)	60 (132)	65 (143)	70 (154)	75 (165)	80 (176)	85 (187)	90 (198)	95 (209)	100 (220)	105 (231)	110 (242)
5	0.42	0.37	0.33	0.30	0.28	0.26	0.24	0.22	0.21	0.20	0.19	0.18	0.17	0.16	0.15
10	0.83	0.74	0.67	0.61	0.56	0.51	0.48	0.44	0.42	0.39	0.37	0.35	0.33	0.32	0.30
15	1.25	1.11	1.00	0.91	0.83	0.77	0.71	0.67	0.63	0.59	0.56	0.53	0.50	0.48	0.45
20	1.67	1.48	1.33	1.21	1.11	1.03	0.95	0.89	0.83	0.78	0.74	0.70	0.67	0.63	0.61
25	2.08	1.85	1.67	1.52	1.39	1.28	1.19	1.11	1.04	0.98	0.93	0.88	0.83	0.79	0.76
30	2.50	2.22	2.00	1.82	1.67	1.54	1.43	1.33	1.25	1.18	1.11	1.05	1.00	0.95	0.91
35	2.92	2.59	2.33	2.12	1.94	1.79	1.67	1.56	1.46	1.37	1.30	1.23	1.17	1.11	1.06
40	3.33	2.96	2.67	2.42	2.22	2.05	1.90	1.78	1.67	1.57	1.48	1.40	1.33	1.27	1.21
45	3.75	3.33	3.00	2.73	2.50	2.31	2.14	2.00	1.88	1.76	1.67	1.58	1.50	1.43	1.36
50	4.17	3.70	3.33	3.03	2.78	2.56	2.38	2.22	2.08	1.96	1.85	1.75	1.67	1.59	1.52
55	4.58	4.07	3.67	3.33	3.06	2.82	2.62	2.44	2.29	2.16	2.04	1.93	1.83	1.75	1.67
60	5.00	4.44	4.00	3.64	3.33	3.08	2.86	2.67	2.50	2.35	2.22	2.11	2.00	1.90	1.82
65	5.42	4.81	4.33	3.94	3.61	3.33	3.10	2.89	2.71	2.55	2.41	2.28	2.17	2.06	1.97
70	5.83	5.19	4.67	4.24	3.89	3.59	3.33	3.11	2.92	2.75	2.59	2.46	2.33	2.22	2.12
75	6.25	5.56	5.00	4.55	4.17	3.85	3.57	3.33	3.13	2.94	2.78	2.63	2.50	2.38	2.27
80	6.67	5.93	5.33	4.85	4.44	4.10	3.81	3.56	3.33	3.14	2.96	2.81	2.67	2.54	2.42
85	7.08	6.30	5.67	5.15	4.72	4.36	4.05	3.78	3.54	3.33	3.15	2.98	2.83	2.70	2.58
90	7.50	6.67	6.00	5.45	5.00	4.62	4.29	4.00	3.75	3.53	3.33	3.16	3.00	2.86	2.73
95	7.92	7.04	6.33	5.76	5.28	4.87	4.52	4.22	3.96	3.73	3.52	3.33	3.17	3.02	2.88
100	8.33	7.41	6.67	6.06	5.56	5.13	4.76	4.44	4.17	3.92	3.70	3.51	3.33	3.17	3.03
105	8.75	7.78	7.00	6.36	5.83	5.38	5.00	4.67	4.38	4.12	3.89	3.68	3.50	3.33	3.18
110	9.17	8.15	7.33	6.67	6.11	5.64	5.24	4.89	4.58	4.31	4.07	3.86	3.67	3.49	3.33
115	9.58	8.52	7.67	6.97	6.39	5.90	5.48	5.11	4.79	4.51	4.26	4.04	3.83	3.65	3.48
120	10.00	8.89	8.00	7.27	6.67	6.15	5.71	5.33	5.00	4.71	4.44	4.21	4.00	3.81	3.64

Morphine Sulfate

Pharmacology

Derivative of opium with agonist effects on neurotransmitter binding and release primarily at kappa and mu receptor sites in the CNS and smooth muscle–containing organs

Principal actions include analgesia via alteration of CNS response to noxious stimuli, peripheral vasodilation, respiratory depression, cough suppression, medulla-induced nausea and vomiting, gastrointestinal hypomotility, increased urinary tract tone, and histamine release

Secondary effects include euphoria, miosis, hypothermia, alterations in consciousness, biliary tract spasm, prolongation of labor, decreased intraocular pressure, hyperglycemia, vasopressin release, and suppressed release of thyroid hormone, corticotropin, and gonadotropins

No significant direct cardiac effects but may cause hypotension

Administrative Guidelines

Administer infusion via precision control device

Carefully monitor ECG and vital signs

Do not use unless emergency resuscitative equipment, trained personnel, and a narcotic antagonist (naloxone) are available

Place patient supine and, if necessary, elevate legs to avoid orthostatic hypotension

Bolus doses should be given slowly over 4–5 minutes to avoid respiratory and circulatory depression

Physical dependence usually not seen until doses exceeding 80 mg for 30 days are employed

Observe for abstinence/withdrawal syndrome

Lipophilic and partially protein bound

Morphine may elevate serum amylase and lipase levels

Contraindicated in those with known hypersensitivity (solutions may contain sodium metabisulfite), upper

(continued below)

Indications

Pain relief in situations in which nonnarcotic analgesics are ineffective during acute myocardial infarction

Adjunct to anesthesia and labor as well as preoperative sedation

Management of pulmonary edema (except in cases in which chemical irritation is causative)

Pharmacokinetics

Onset of Action. 7–20 minutes after IV bolus

Peak Effects. Within 20 minutes after IV bolus

Duration of Action. Up to 7 hours

Tissue (Elimination) Half-Life. 1.5–2 hours

Metabolism. Via liver conjugation with glucuronic acid and primarily urinary excretion

airway obstruction, acute bronchospasm, or diarrhea induced by poisoning until the toxin has cleared

Use with caution in patients with toxic psychosis; geriatric or debilitated patients; those with a history of drug abuse or dependence; those with renal or hepatic dysfunction, respiratory depression, chronic obstructive lung disease, hypotension, depressed myocardial function, elevated intraocular or intracranial pressure, head injury or intracranial pathology; and those taking sympatholytics

Exercise extreme caution and consider reducing dose in patients with ulcerative colitis, biliary colic, Addison's disease, hypothyroidism, prostatic hypertrophy, urinary retention, CNS depression, anoxia, and hypercapnia; those prone to respiratory depression, fever, urethral stricture, severe obesity, shock, cor pulmonale, emphysema, myxedema, acute alcohol intoxication and delirium tremens, kyphoscoliosis, and tachydysrhythmias; in patients performing tasks requiring mental acuity; and in patients with tartrazine sensitivity

(continued on page 186)

Overdosage may manifest with respiratory depression and hypotension. Manage with supportive and symptomatic measures and establishment of adequate ventilation. Consider naloxone hydrochloride 0.4–2.0 mg IV every 2–3 minutes to a total dose of 10 mg. Continuous infusions of 0.0037 mg/kg/hr may be used to combat postoperative respiratory depression

Dosing Information

IV Bolus. 2–10 mg (0.03–0.15 mg/kg) **diluted** in 4–5 mL sterile water given over 4–5 minutes

Initial Infusion Dose. 1–10 mg/hr

Maintenance Infusion Range. 20–150 mg/hr

Maximum Infusion Rate. 150 mg/hr

Titration Guideline

Suggested Regimen

IV Bolus. Repeat 2–10 mg (0.03–0.15 mg/kg) every 3–4 hours as necessary

IV Infusion. Adjust infusion by 1–10 mg/hr every 30–60 minutes as necessary

Potential Drug Interactions

Potentiation of Morphine Effects. General anesthetics, phenothiazines, antihistamines, opiate agonists, barbiturates, sedative hypnotics, tricyclic and other antidepressants, alcohol, chlorpromazine, chloral hydrate, glutethimide, beta-adrenergic blockers, methocarbamol, furazolidone, and possibly cimetidine

Antagonism of Morphine Effects. Naloxone, phenothiazines

Possibly Potentiated by Morphine. Diuretics in patients with congestive heart failure

Morphine Sulfate

How Supplied

IV Injection

0.5 mg/mL—2-mL ampuls and vials of 1 mg; 10-mL ampuls and vials of 5 mg

1.0 mg/mL—2-mL ampuls of 2 mg; 10-mL ampuls and vials of 10 mg; 30-mL ampuls of 30 mg; 60-mL ampuls of 60 mg

2.0 mg/mL—1-mL syringe (Tubex) of 2 mg; 2-mL syringe (Tubex) of 4 mg; 6-mL vials of 12 mg

3.0 mg/mL—50-mL vials of 150 mg

4.0 mg/mL—1-mL syringe (Tubex) of 4 mg; 2-mL syringe (Tubex) of 8 mg

5.0 mg/mL—1-mL vial of 5 mg; 30-mL vials of 150 mg

8.0 mg/mL—1-mL vials, ampuls, and syringes (Tubex) of 8 mg; 2-mL syringes (Tubex) of 16 mg

10 mg/mL—1-mL ampuls, vials, and syringes (Tubex) of 10 mg; 2-mL syringes (Tubex) of 20 mg; 10-mL vials of 100 mg

(continued below)

Principal Adverse Effects

CNS. Altered mental status, coma, headache, miosis, anxiety, insomnia, tremor, weakness, visual disturbances, dizziness, lightheadedness, and agitation

Pulmonary. Respiratory depression, apnea, arrest

CV. Hypotension, syncope, shock, bradycardia, tachycardia, hypertension, cardiac arrest, orthostasis

GI. Nausea, vomiting, anorexia, dry mouth, constipation, biliary spasm, toxic bowel dilation in ulcerative colitis

GU. Decreased libido, urinary retention, ureteral spasm, antidiuresis

Allergic. Anaphylactoid reactions, flushing, rash, diaphoresis, edema, pruritus, thrombocytopenia

15 mg/mL—1-mL ampuls, vials, and syringes (Tubex) of 15 mg; 2-mL syringes of 30 mg; 20-mL ampuls and vials of 300 mg

IV Infusion

1 mg/mL—10-, 30-, 50-, and 60-mL preparations

2 mg/mL—60-mL preparation of 120 mg

3 mg/mL—50-mL preparation of 150 mg

5 mg/mL—30-mL preparation of 150 mg

10 mg/mL—3-mL (30 mg) and 6-mL (60 mg) preparations

25 mg/mL—4-mL (100 mg), 10-mL (250 mg), 20-mL (500 mg), and 40-mL (1000 mg) preparations

50 mg/mL—10-mL (500 mg), 20-mL (1000 mg), and 40-mL (2000 mg) preparations

Morphine Sulfate

250 mg in 500 mL

■ Infusion Rate in mL/hr (pump setting) ■ Drug Dose in mg/hr

1	0.5	21	10.5	41	20.5	61	30.5	81	40.5	101	50.5
2	1.0	22	11.0	42	21.0	62	31.0	82	41.0	102	51.0
3	1.5	23	11.5	43	21.5	63	31.5	83	41.5	103	51.5
4	2.0	24	12.0	44	22.0	64	32.0	84	42.0	104	52.0
5	2.5	25	12.5	45	22.5	65	32.5	85	42.5	105	52.5
6	3.0	26	13.0	46	23.0	66	33.0	86	43.0	106	53.0
7	3.5	27	13.5	47	23.5	67	33.5	87	43.5	107	53.5
8	4.0	28	14.0	48	24.0	68	34.0	88	44.0	108	54.0
9	4.5	29	14.5	49	24.5	69	34.5	89	44.5	109	54.5
10	5.0	30	15.0	50	25.0	70	35.0	90	45.0	110	55.0
11	5.5	31	15.5	51	25.5	71	35.5	91	45.5	111	55.5
12	6.0	32	16.0	52	26.0	72	36.0	92	46.0	112	56.0
13	6.5	33	16.5	53	26.5	73	36.5	93	46.5	113	56.5
14	7.0	34	17.0	54	27.0	74	37.0	94	47.0	114	57.0
15	7.5	35	17.5	55	27.5	75	37.5	95	47.5	115	57.5
16	8.0	36	18.0	56	28.0	76	38.0	96	48.0	116	58.0
17	8.5	37	18.5	57	28.5	77	38.5	97	48.5	117	58.5
18	9.0	38	19.0	58	29.0	78	39.0	98	49.0	118	59.0
19	9.5	39	19.5	59	29.5	79	39.5	99	49.5	119	59.5
20	10.0	40	20.0	60	30.0	80	40.0	100	50.0	120	60.0

■ Infusion Rate in mL/hr (pump setting) ■ Drug Dose in mg/hr

mL/hr	mg/hr	mL/hr	mg/hr	mL/hr	mg/hr	mL/hr	mg/hr	mL/hr	mg/hr	mL/hr	mg/hr
1	1.0	21	21.0	41	41.0	61	61.0	81	81.0	101	101.0
2	2.0	22	22.0	42	42.0	62	62.0	82	82.0	102	102.0
3	3.0	23	23.0	43	43.0	63	63.0	83	83.0	103	103.0
4	4.0	24	24.0	44	44.0	64	64.0	84	84.0	104	104.0
5	5.0	25	25.0	45	45.0	65	65.0	85	85.0	105	105.0
6	6.0	26	26.0	46	46.0	66	66.0	86	86.0	106	106.0
7	7.0	27	27.0	47	47.0	67	67.0	87	87.0	107	107.0
8	8.0	28	28.0	48	48.0	68	68.0	88	88.0	108	108.0
9	9.0	29	29.0	49	49.0	69	69.0	89	89.0	109	109.0
10	10.0	30	30.0	50	50.0	70	70.0	90	90.0	110	110.0
11	11.0	31	31.0	51	51.0	71	71.0	91	91.0	111	111.0
12	12.0	32	32.0	52	52.0	72	72.0	92	92.0	112	112.0
13	13.0	33	33.0	53	53.0	73	73.0	93	93.0	113	113.0
14	14.0	34	34.0	54	54.0	74	74.0	94	94.0	114	114.0
15	15.0	35	35.0	55	55.0	75	75.0	95	95.0	115	115.0
16	16.0	36	36.0	56	56.0	76	76.0	96	96.0	116	116.0
17	17.0	37	37.0	57	57.0	77	77.0	97	97.0	117	117.0
18	18.0	38	38.0	58	58.0	78	78.0	98	98.0	118	118.0
19	19.0	39	39.0	59	59.0	79	79.0	99	99.0	119	119.0
20	20.0	40	40.0	60	60.0	80	80.0	100	100.0	120	120.0

Naloxone Hydrochloride (Narcan)

Pharmacology

Semisynthetic opiate antagonist with no significant narcotic agonist properties

Mechanism of action thought to be competitive block of mu, kappa, and sigma opiate receptors in the CNS

Reverses respiratory depression, sedation, and hypotension produced by morphine and other opiate cogeners

Does not cause physical or psychological dependence or tolerance

Virtually no pharmacologic effects when administered to patients who have not received opiates

Administrative Guidelines

Administer infusion via precision control device

Carefully monitor ECG and vital signs

Do not mix with alkaline solutions or preparations containing bisulfites, metabisulfites, or long-chain/high-molecular-weight anions

May be administered intramuscularly, subcutaneously, or probably by endotracheal tube if IV access not available

Avoid excessive dose postoperatively to prevent clinically detrimental excitatory states, nausea, vomiting, sweating, and tachycardia

Observe treated patients for return of opiate effects because naloxone has shorter duration of action than that of most narcotics

Naloxone is not effective in reversing respiratory depression secondary to nonopioid drugs

Contraindicated with known hypersensitivity

(continued below)

Indications

Treatment and reversal of narcotic-induced respiratory depression

Diagnosis of suspected acute opiate overdosage

Unlabeled Uses. To combat emetic effects and respiratory depression induced by apomorphine; to detect chronic opiate abuse; to reverse coma secondary to clonidine or alcohol; to treat septic shock, cardiogenic shock, high altitude pulmonary edema, acute respiratory failure, senile dementia, and ischemic neurologic deficits

Pharmacokinetics

Onset of Action. 1–2 minutes

Peak Effects. Within 45 minutes

Duration of Action. Approximately 45 minutes

Metabolism. Via liver with excretion by the kidney

Use with caution in patients with known or suspected opiate physical dependence (may produce withdrawal symptoms), those receiving cardiotoxic drugs, or those with preexisting cardiovascular disease (may precipitate life-threatening ventricular dysrhythmias)

Overdosage management has not been established in humans

Naloxone Hydrochloride (Narcan)

Dosing Information

Known or Suspected Narcotic Overdosage

IV Bolus Regimen. 0.4–2.0 mg. May repeat at 2- to 3-minute intervals up to 10 mg

IV Infusion Regimen. 0.4 mg IV load, then 0.4 mg per hour or 0.005 mg/kg IV load, then 0.0025 mg/kg per hour

Postoperative Narcotic Depression

IV Bolus Regimen. 0.1–0.2 mg. Repeat at 2- to 3-minute intervals until desired response noted. May repeat regimen at 1 to 2 hour intervals as necessary or 0.005 mg/kg IV bolus. May repeat at 15-minute intervals as necessary

IV Infusion Regimen. 0.0037 mg/kg/hr

Maximum Infusion Range. Not specified by manufacturer.

Potential Drug Interactions

Possibly Antagonized by Naloxone. Opiates

Principal Adverse Effects

CNS. Irritability, drowsiness, depression, apathy, tremulousness, seizures, diaphoresis, hyperventilation

CV. Ventricular tachycardia and fibrillation, hypertension, hypotension, pulmonary edema

GI. Nausea, vomiting, anorexia

Miscellaneous. Erythema multiforme

How Supplied

0.4 mg/mL—1-mL ampuls, syringes, and vials of 0.4 mg
2-mL vials of 0.8 mg
10-mL vials of 4 mg

1.0 mg/mL—2-mL ampuls and vials of 2 mg
10-mL vials of 10 mg

Naloxone Hydrochloride (Narcan) 4 mg in 500 mL

■ Infusion Rate in mL/hr (pump setting) ■ Drug Dose in mg/hr

mL/hr	mg/hr	mL/hr	mg/hr	mL/hr	mg/hr	mL/hr	mg/hr	mL/hr	mg/hr	mL/hr	mg/hr
1	0.008	21	0.168	41	0.328	61	0.488	81	0.648	101	0.808
2	0.016	22	0.176	42	0.336	62	0.496	82	0.656	102	0.816
3	0.024	23	0.184	43	0.344	63	0.504	83	0.664	103	0.824
4	0.032	24	0.192	44	0.352	64	0.512	84	0.672	104	0.832
5	0.040	25	0.200	45	0.360	65	0.520	85	0.680	105	0.840
6	0.048	26	0.208	46	0.368	66	0.528	86	0.688	106	0.848
7	0.056	27	0.216	47	0.376	67	0.536	87	0.696	107	0.856
8	0.064	28	0.224	48	0.384	68	0.544	88	0.704	108	0.864
9	0.072	29	0.232	49	0.392	69	0.552	89	0.712	109	0.872
10	0.080	30	0.240	50	0.400	70	0.560	90	0.720	110	0.880
11	0.088	31	0.248	51	0.408	71	0.568	91	0.728	111	0.888
12	0.096	32	0.256	52	0.416	72	0.576	92	0.736	112	0.896
13	0.104	33	0.264	53	0.424	73	0.584	93	0.744	113	0.904
14	0.112	34	0.272	54	0.432	74	0.592	94	0.752	114	0.912
15	0.120	35	0.280	55	0.440	75	0.600	95	0.760	115	0.920
16	0.128	36	0.288	56	0.448	76	0.608	96	0.768	116	0.928
17	0.136	37	0.296	57	0.456	77	0.616	97	0.776	117	0.936
18	0.144	38	0.304	58	0.464	78	0.624	98	0.784	118	0.944
19	0.152	39	0.312	59	0.472	79	0.632	99	0.792	119	0.952
20	0.160	40	0.320	60	0.480	80	0.640	100	0.800	120	0.960

DRUG DOSE in mg/kg/hr

Patient's Weight

Infusion Rate in mL/hr	kg 40 / lbs 88	kg 45 / lbs 99	kg 50 / lbs 110	kg 55 / lbs 121	kg 60 / lbs 132	kg 65 / lbs 143	kg 70 / lbs 154	kg 75 / lbs 165	kg 80 / lbs 176	kg 85 / lbs 187	kg 90 / lbs 198	kg 95 / lbs 209	kg 100 / lbs 220	kg 105 / lbs 231	kg 110 / lbs 242
5	0.0010	0.0009	0.0008	0.0007	0.0007	0.0006	0.0006	0.0005	0.0005	0.0005	0.0004	0.0004	0.0004	0.0004	0.0004
10	0.0020	0.0018	0.0016	0.0015	0.0013	0.0012	0.0011	0.0011	0.0010	0.0009	0.0009	0.0008	0.0008	0.0008	0.0007
15	0.0030	0.0027	0.0024	0.0022	0.0020	0.0018	0.0017	0.0016	0.0015	0.0014	0.0013	0.0013	0.0012	0.0011	0.0011
20	0.0040	0.0036	0.0032	0.0029	0.0027	0.0025	0.0023	0.0021	0.0020	0.0019	0.0018	0.0017	0.0016	0.0015	0.0015
25	0.0050	0.0044	0.0040	0.0036	0.0033	0.0031	0.0029	0.0027	0.0025	0.0024	0.0022	0.0021	0.0020	0.0019	0.0018
30	0.0060	0.0053	0.0048	0.0044	0.0040	0.0037	0.0034	0.0032	0.0030	0.0028	0.0027	0.0025	0.0024	0.0023	0.0022
35	0.0070	0.0062	0.0056	0.0051	0.0047	0.0043	0.0040	0.0037	0.0035	0.0033	0.0031	0.0029	0.0028	0.0027	0.0025
40	0.0080	0.0071	0.0064	0.0058	0.0053	0.0049	0.0046	0.0043	0.0040	0.0038	0.0036	0.0034	0.0032	0.0030	0.0029
45	0.0090	0.0080	0.0072	0.0065	0.0060	0.0055	0.0051	0.0048	0.0045	0.0042	0.0040	0.0038	0.0036	0.0034	0.0033
50	0.0100	0.0089	0.0080	0.0073	0.0067	0.0062	0.0057	0.0053	0.0050	0.0047	0.0044	0.0042	0.0040	0.0038	0.0036
55	0.0110	0.0098	0.0088	0.0080	0.0073	0.0068	0.0063	0.0059	0.0055	0.0052	0.0049	0.0046	0.0044	0.0042	0.0040
60	0.0120	0.0107	0.0096	0.0087	0.0080	0.0074	0.0069	0.0064	0.0060	0.0056	0.0053	0.0051	0.0048	0.0046	0.0044
65	0.0130	0.0116	0.0104	0.0095	0.0087	0.0080	0.0074	0.0069	0.0065	0.0061	0.0058	0.0055	0.0052	0.0050	0.0047
70	0.0140	0.0124	0.0112	0.0102	0.0093	0.0086	0.0080	0.0075	0.0070	0.0066	0.0062	0.0059	0.0056	0.0053	0.0051
75	0.0150	0.0133	0.0120	0.0109	0.0100	0.0092	0.0086	0.0080	0.0075	0.0071	0.0067	0.0063	0.0060	0.0057	0.0055
80	0.0160	0.0142	0.0128	0.0116	0.0107	0.0098	0.0091	0.0085	0.0080	0.0075	0.0071	0.0067	0.0064	0.0061	0.0058
85	0.0170	0.0151	0.0136	0.0124	0.0113	0.0105	0.0097	0.0091	0.0085	0.0080	0.0076	0.0072	0.0068	0.0065	0.0062
90	0.0180	0.0160	0.0144	0.0131	0.0120	0.0111	0.0103	0.0096	0.0090	0.0085	0.0080	0.0076	0.0072	0.0069	0.0065
95	0.0190	0.0169	0.0152	0.0138	0.0127	0.0117	0.0109	0.0101	0.0095	0.0089	0.0084	0.0080	0.0076	0.0072	0.0069
100	0.0200	0.0178	0.0160	0.0145	0.0133	0.0123	0.0114	0.0107	0.0100	0.0094	0.0089	0.0084	0.0080	0.0076	0.0073
105	0.0210	0.0187	0.0168	0.0153	0.0140	0.0129	0.0120	0.0112	0.0105	0.0099	0.0093	0.0088	0.0084	0.0080	0.0076
110	0.0220	0.0196	0.0176	0.0160	0.0147	0.0135	0.0126	0.0117	0.0110	0.0104	0.0098	0.0093	0.0088	0.0084	0.0080
115	0.0230	0.0204	0.0184	0.0167	0.0153	0.0142	0.0131	0.0123	0.0115	0.0108	0.0102	0.0097	0.0092	0.0088	0.0084
120	0.0240	0.0213	0.0192	0.0175	0.0160	0.0148	0.0137	0.0128	0.0120	0.0113	0.0107	0.0101	0.0096	0.0091	0.0087

Nitroglycerin (Nitrostat, Tridil)

Pharmacology

Produces relaxation of vascular smooth muscle by stimulating intracellular cyclic guanosine monophosphate production

Primarily affects venous (capacitance) vessels with some reduction in arteriolar (resistance) vessel tone in a dose-dependent manner

Relaxes all vascular smooth muscle beds regardless of autonomic innervation and functionally antagonizes histamine, acetylcholine, and norepinephrine

Decreases myocardial oxygen consumption by reducing preload, afterload, and ventricular wall tension—variable effects on cardiac output

May reflexly increase heart rate and contractility

Reduces systemic vascular resistance and pressure and lowers pulmonary vascular resistance and pressure

Variable effects on total coronary blood flow with coronary perfusion pressure usually preserved

(continued below)

Administrative Guidelines

Administer infusion via precision control device

Monitor ECG continuously, and carefully follow blood pressure, vital signs, and, if available, hemodynamic measurements

Correct any underlying hypovolemia, if possible, before use, and observe for postural hypotension

Nitroglycerin is readily absorbed by plastics and some IV filters. 40–80% of infused nitroglycerin may be absorbed into polyvinyl chloride (PVC) tubing or bags. Prepare infusion solution in glass bottles, employ non-PVC administration sets, and avoid IV filters

Tachyphylaxis to nitrates may occur rapidly, especially with higher doses. Employ smallest effective dose, avoid escalating infusion rate, and consider nitrate-free period

Cross-tolerance to other nitrate preparations and drug dependence rarely, if ever, develops

(continued below)

May improve perfusion to ischemic myocardium by redistributing coronary blood flow via collateral vessel effects, dilating conductance vessels, and enhancing subendocardial blood supply

May increase urinary catecholamines by activating adrenergic receptors secondary to hypotensive actions

Indications

Management of uncontrolled hypertension, including that associated with cardiovascular procedures and coronary complications

Control of blood pressure during surgical interventions

Treatment of angina pectoris in those who have not responded to nitrates and beta-blockers

Ischemic pain and congestive heart failure associated with acute myocardial infarction

Unlabeled Uses. Hypertensive crises, refractory heart failure, low cardiac output states, and limiting ischemia and infarct size during acute myocardial infarction

Alcohol intoxication may ensue with prolonged use because alcohol is a commercial additive to infusion solution

Nitroglycerin may falsely decrease serum cholesterol measurement

Contraindicated with known hypersensitivity, severe anemia, head trauma, cerebral hemorrhage, increased intracranial pressure, uncorrected hypovolemia, hypotension, and pericardial constriction or tamponade

Use with caution in glaucoma, acute myocardial infarction, gastrointestinal hypermotility or malabsorption syndromes, hypertrophic cardiomyopathy, diuretic-induced hypovolemia, or systolic blood pressure below 90 mmHg

Overdosage typically produces signs and symptoms of vasodilation, including hypotension, headache, tachycardia, diaphoresis, and confusion. Manage with fluids, supportive measures, and alpha-adrenergic agents in extreme cases. Epinephrine is ineffective and contraindicated for hypotension

(continued on page 200)

Nitroglycerin (Nitrostat, Tridil)

Pharmacokinetics

Onset of Action. 1–2 minutes

Peak Effects. 1–5 minutes

Duration of Action. 3–5 minutes

Plasma (Distribution) Half-Life. 1–4 minutes

Metabolism. Via liver by nitrate reductase with production of active metabolites

Methemoglobinemia is also possible secondary to overdosage and manifests with cyanosis, acidosis, vomiting, shock, seizures, and coma. Manage with supportive measures, high-flow oxygen, and 1–2 mg/kg methylene blue by slow IV push

Dosing Information

Initial Infusion Rate. 5–10 μg/min

Maintenance Infusion Range. 5–100 μg/min

Maximum Infusion Rate. Not specified by manufacturer but doses beyond 400 μg/min are rarely indicated

Titration Guideline

Suggested Regimen. Adjust infusion by 5–10 μg/min every 3–5 minutes as required

How Supplied

IV Injection

0.5 mg/mL—10-mL ampuls of 5 mg

0.8 mg/mL—10-mL ampuls of 8 mg

5 mg/mL—1-mL vials of 5 mg
5-mL vials and ampuls of 25 mg
10-mL vials and ampuls of 50 mg
20-mL vials of 100 mg

(continued on page 202)

Potential Drug Interactions

Potentiation of Nitroglycerin Effects. Alcohol, aspirin, calcium channel blockers, beta-blockers, antihypertensive agents, phenothiazines

Antagonism of Nitroglycerin Effects. Dihydroergotamine

Possibly Antagonized by Nitroglycerin. Heparin

Nitroglycerin (Nitrostat, Tridil)

Premixed IV Infusion

100 μg/mL—25 mg in 250 mL 5% dextrose
50 mg in 500 mL 5% dextrose

200 μg/mL—50 mg in 250 mL 5% dextrose

400 μg/mL—100 mg in 250 mL 5% dextrose
200 mg in 500 mL 5% dextrose

Principal Adverse Effects

CNS. Headache, weakness, vertigo, apprehension, flushing, insomnia, dizziness, anxiety, confusion, nightmares, muscle twitching and incoordination, and agitation

Pulmonary. Bronchitis, pneumonia, wheezing, and tracheitis

CV. Hypotension, bradycardia, tachycardia, heart block, hypertension, syncope, angina, palpitations, atrial and ventricular dysrhythmias, and shock

GI. Nausea, vomiting, abdominal pain, incontinence, tenesmus, diarrhea, and dyspepsia

GU. Dysuria, impotence, urinary frequency

Dermatological. Rash, pruritus

Musculoskeletal. Myalgia

Miscellaneous. Methemoglobinemia, pallor, hemolytic anemia, diplopia, blurred vision, asthenia, edema, malaise, rigors, neck stiffness, increased appetite

Nitroglycerin (Nitrostat, Tridil)

50 mg in 250 mL

■ **Infusion Rate in mL/hr (pump setting)** ■ **Drug Dose in μg/min**

mL/hr	μg/min	mL/hr	μg/min	mL/hr	μg/min	mL/hr	μg/min	mL/hr	μg/min	mL/hr	μg/min
1	3	21	70	41	137	61	203	81	270	101	337
2	7	22	73	42	140	62	207	82	273	102	340
3	10	23	77	43	143	63	210	83	277	103	343
4	13	24	80	44	147	64	213	84	280	104	347
5	17	25	83	45	150	65	217	85	283	105	350
6	20	26	87	46	153	66	220	86	287	106	353
7	23	27	90	47	157	67	223	87	290	107	357
8	27	28	93	48	160	68	227	88	293	108	360
9	30	29	97	49	163	69	230	89	297	109	363
10	33	30	100	50	167	70	233	90	300	110	367
11	37	31	103	51	170	71	237	91	303	111	370
12	40	32	107	52	173	72	240	92	307	112	373
13	43	33	110	53	177	73	243	93	310	113	377
14	47	34	113	54	180	74	247	94	313	114	380
15	50	35	117	55	183	75	250	95	317	115	383
16	53	36	120	56	187	76	253	96	320	116	387
17	57	37	123	57	190	77	257	97	323	117	390
18	60	38	127	58	193	78	260	98	327	118	393
19	63	39	130	59	197	79	263	99	330	119	397
20	67	40	133	60	200	80	267	100	333	120	400

■ Infusion Rate in mL/hr (pump setting) ■ Drug Dose in µg/min

Infusion Rate	Drug Dose	Infusion Rate	Drug Dose	Infusion Rate	Drug Dose	Infusion Rate	Drug Dose	Infusion Rate	Drug Dose	Infusion Rate	Drug Dose
1	7	21	140	41	273	61	407	81	540	101	673
2	13	22	147	42	280	62	413	82	547	102	680
3	20	23	153	43	287	63	420	83	553	103	687
4	27	24	160	44	293	64	427	84	560	104	693
5	33	25	167	45	300	65	433	85	567	105	700
6	40	26	173	46	307	66	440	86	573	106	707
7	47	27	180	47	313	67	447	87	580	107	713
8	53	28	187	48	320	68	453	88	587	108	720
9	60	29	193	49	327	69	460	89	593	109	727
10	67	30	200	50	333	70	467	90	600	110	733
11	73	31	207	51	340	71	473	91	607	111	740
12	80	32	213	52	347	72	480	92	613	112	747
13	87	33	220	53	353	73	487	93	620	113	753
14	93	34	227	54	360	74	493	94	627	114	760
15	100	35	233	55	367	75	500	95	633	115	767
16	107	36	240	56	373	76	507	96	640	116	773
17	113	37	247	57	380	77	513	97	647	117	780
18	120	38	253	58	387	78	520	98	653	118	787
19	127	39	260	59	393	79	527	99	660	119	793
20	133	40	267	60	400	80	533	100	667	120	800

Norepinephrine Bitartrate (Levophed)

Pharmacology

Endogenous catecholamine (L-isomer) produced by the adrenal medulla and sympathetic neurons, which stimulates both alpha- and beta-adrenergic receptors

Alpha- and beta-adrenergic effects are mediated by inhibition and activation of adenyl cyclase (influences cyclic adenosine monophosphate production)

Alpha effects predominate with vasoconstriction of resistance and capacitance vessels. Increases systemic pressure and pulmonary vascular resistance and pressure. Blood flow to vital organs, skeletal muscle, skin, uterus, kidneys, and cerebrum is usually reduced. Hypotensive patients, however, may experience augmented cerebral, renal, and coronary blood flow. Postcapillary vasoconstriction may promote extracellular fluid loss and reduced plasma volume (especially with prolonged use)

Direct $beta_1$ stimulation also noted, but this response is less potent than with epinephrine or isoproterenol. Positive inotropic action may augment cardiac output

(continued below)

Administrative Guidelines

Administer infusion via precision control device

Continuously monitor vital signs, ECG, and renal function—carefully follow acid-base status and, if available, hemodynamic variables

Administer via central line, if possible, or large antecubital vein—avoid infusing through cut-down site

Always dilute before use—recommend 5% dextrose injection USP to prevent oxidation and loss of potency

Discard solution if brown, pink, or dark yellow discoloration is noted or precipitate observed

Do not admix with blood or plasma, sodium bicarbonate, iron salts, barbiturates, alkaline solutions or antibiotics, and oxidizing agents

Do not use as sole treatment in patients with hypovolemia

Correct electrolyte abnormalities, acid-base status, and volume depletion, if possible, before use or concurrently with therapy

(continued below)

and myocardial oxygen consumption. Positive chronotropic action on sinoatrial node is usually offset by reflex vagal response secondary to increased blood pressure. Cardiac tachydysrhythmias are occasionally noted

No significant $beta_2$ effects on peripheral blood vessels or bronchi

Respiratory stimulation does not occur, but brief apnea may develop

Norepinephrine can increase glycogenolysis; inhibit insulin release; enhance lipolysis, free fatty acid concentration, lactic acid, and cholesterol levels; and elevate total body oxygen consumption and temperature

Closely observe infusion site for free-flow, blanching, and extravasation

Extravasation requires discontinuation of infusion and immediate subcutaneous infiltration of 5–10 mg phentolamine mesylate in 10–15 mL normal saline (effective up to 12 hours following extravasation). Consider adding 100–200 units heparin or 5–10 mg phentolamine to infusion of norepinephrine as prophylaxis against perivascular reaction, thrombosis, and skin sloughing

Contraindicated in those with known hypersensitivity, profound hypercapnia; or hypoxia; as sole therapy in hypovolemic patients; during cyclopropane or halogenated hydrocarbon anesthesia; and in those with mesenteric or peripheral vascular thrombosis

Use with caution in patients with suspected sulfite sensitivity (contains sodium metabisulfite); those with hypertension or hyperthyroidism or occlusive vascular disease; or in patients using tricyclic antidepressants, monoamine oxidase inhibitors, antihistamines, methyldopa, guanethidine, and parenteral ergot alkaloids

(continued on page 208)

Norepinephrine Bitartrate (Levophed)

Indications

Short-term support of blood pressure and cardiac stimulation in nonhypovolemic shock; management of hypotension during spinal or general anesthesia; adjunctive therapy to augment perfusion during cardiopulmonary arrest

Unlabeled Use. Cardiac tamponade associated with hypotension and depressed cardiac output

Pharmacokinetics

Onset of Action. Within 1–2 minutes

Peak Effects. 1–2 minutes

Duration of Action. 1–2 minutes

Metabolism. Via liver and sympathetic nerve endings to inactive metabolites

Overdosage may manifest with severe hypertension, reflex bradycardia, marked peripheral vasoconstriction, and reduced cardiac output. Manage with supportive measures and appropriate fluid and electrolyte correction

Dosing Information

Initial Infusion Rate

During Advanced Cardiac Life Support. 0.5–1.0 μg/min

Severe Hypotension. 8–12 μg/min

Maintenance Infusion Rate. 2–4 μg/min

Maximal Infusion Rate. Rarely greater than 47 μg/min

Maximal Daily Dose. 68 mg

Dosages are expressed in milligrams of norepinephrine (1 mg of norepinephrine is equivalent to 2 mg of norepinephrine bitartrate)

Titration Guideline

Suggested Regimen. Adjust infusion by 1–2 μg/min every 2 minutes as necessary for blood pressure control

How Supplied

1 mg/mL—4-mL ampuls of 4 mg

Potential Drug Interactions

Potentiation of Norepinephrine Effects. Monoamine oxidase inhibitors, tricyclic antidepressants, guanethidine, methyldopa, parenteral ergot alkaloids, antihistamines, atropine, oxytocic agents, cyclopropane or halogenated hydrocarbon anesthetics, digitalis glycosides

Antagonism of Norepinephrine Effects. Beta-blockers, thiazide diuretics, furosemide

Norepinephrine Bitartrate (Levophed)

Principal Adverse Effects

CNS. Headache, restlessness, tremor, weakness, dizziness, anxiety, insomnia, cerebral hemorrhage, convulsions, and photophobia

Pulmonary. Respiratory distress, apnea

CV. Hypertension, reflex bradycardia, hypervolemia, increased peripheral resistance, decreased cardiac output, splanchnic and renal vasoconstriction, tissue hypoxia, lactic acidosis, dysrhythmias, chest pain, palpitations

GI. Vomiting

Dermatological. Sloughing and necrosis of skin at the infusion site, gangrene of extremities

Miscellaneous. Thyroid and pharyngeal pain, pallor

Norepinephrine Bitartrate (Levophed) 8 mg in 500 mL

■ **Infusion Rate in mL/hr (pump setting)** ■ **Drug Dose in μg/min**

mL/hr	μg/min	mL/hr	μg/min	mL/hr	μg/min	mL/hr	μg/min	mL/hr	μg/min	mL/hr	μg/min
1	0.3	21	5.6	41	10.9	61	16.3	81	21.6	101	26.9
2	0.5	22	5.9	42	11.2	62	16.5	82	21.9	102	27.2
3	0.8	23	6.1	43	11.5	63	16.8	83	22.1	103	27.5
4	1.1	24	6.4	44	11.7	64	17.1	84	22.4	104	27.7
5	1.3	25	6.7	45	12.0	65	17.3	85	22.7	105	28.0
6	1.6	26	6.9	46	12.3	66	17.6	86	22.9	106	28.3
7	1.9	27	7.2	47	12.5	67	17.9	87	23.2	107	28.5
8	2.1	28	7.5	48	12.8	68	18.1	88	23.5	108	28.8
9	2.4	29	7.7	49	13.1	69	18.4	89	23.7	109	29.1
10	2.7	30	8.0	50	13.3	70	18.7	90	24.0	110	29.3
11	2.9	31	8.3	51	13.6	71	18.9	91	24.3	111	29.6
12	3.2	32	8.5	52	13.9	72	19.2	92	24.5	112	29.9
13	3.5	33	8.8	53	14.1	73	19.5	93	24.8	113	30.1
14	3.7	34	9.1	54	14.4	74	19.7	94	25.1	114	30.4
15	4.0	35	9.3	55	14.7	75	20.0	95	25.3	115	30.7
16	4.3	36	9.6	56	14.9	76	20.3	96	25.6	116	30.9
17	4.5	37	9.9	57	15.2	77	20.5	97	25.9	117	31.2
18	4.8	38	10.1	58	15.5	78	20.8	98	26.1	118	31.5
19	5.1	39	10.4	59	15.7	79	21.1	99	26.4	119	31.7
20	5.3	40	10.7	60	16.0	80	21.3	100	26.7	120	32.0

Norepinephrine Bitartrate (Levophed) 8 mg in 250 mL

■ Infusion Rate in mL/hr (pump setting) ■ Drug Dose in µg/min

mL/hr	µg/min	mL/hr	µg/min	mL/hr	µg/min	mL/hr	µg/min	mL/hr	µg/min	mL/hr	µg/min
1	0.5	21	11.2	41	21.9	61	32.5	81	43.2	101	53.9
2	1.1	22	11.7	42	22.4	62	33.1	82	43.7	102	54.4
3	1.6	23	12.3	43	22.9	63	33.6	83	44.3	103	54.9
4	2.1	24	12.8	44	23.5	64	34.1	84	44.8	104	55.5
5	2.7	25	13.3	45	24.0	65	34.7	85	45.3	105	56.0
6	3.2	26	13.9	46	24.5	66	35.2	86	45.9	106	56.5
7	3.7	27	14.4	47	25.1	67	35.7	87	46.4	107	57.1
8	4.3	28	14.9	48	25.6	68	36.3	88	46.9	108	57.6
9	4.8	29	15.5	49	26.1	69	36.8	89	47.5	109	58.1
10	5.3	30	16.0	50	26.7	70	37.3	90	48.0	110	58.7
11	5.9	31	16.5	51	27.2	71	37.9	91	48.5	111	59.2
12	6.4	32	17.1	52	27.7	72	38.4	92	49.1	112	59.7
13	6.9	33	17.6	53	28.3	73	38.9	93	49.6	113	60.3
14	7.5	34	18.1	54	28.8	74	39.5	94	50.1	114	60.8
15	8.0	35	18.7	55	29.3	75	40.0	95	50.7	115	61.3
16	8.5	36	19.2	56	29.9	76	40.5	96	51.2	116	61.9
17	9.1	37	19.7	57	30.4	77	41.1	97	51.7	117	62.4
18	9.6	38	20.3	58	30.9	78	41.6	98	52.3	118	62.9
19	10.1	39	20.8	59	31.5	79	42.1	99	52.8	119	63.5
20	10.7	40	21.3	60	32.0	80	42.7	100	53.3	120	64.0

Pancuronium Bromide (Pavulon)

Pharmacology

Synthetic nondepolarizing neuromuscular blocker that competes for cholinergic receptors at the motor end plate

Produces skeletal muscle paralysis via reduced acetylcholine responsiveness at the myoneural junction

May increase heart rate by direct blocking effect on acetylcholine cardiac receptors

Histamine release is rare, and no significant ganglionic blockade is evident

Alteration in consciousness, pain threshold, or cerebration does not occur

Potency is five times greater than *d*-tubocurarine but one-third that of vecuronium

Administrative Guidelines

Administer infusion via precision control device

Monitor ECG, respiration, and blood pressure continuously

Do not administer unless oxygen, anticholinesterase reversal agents, endotracheal intubation equipment, mechanical ventilation, and skilled personnel are in attendance

Avoid infusion through the same site with alkaline solutions or barbiturates

Carefully monitor adductor pollicis muscle with twitch response to peripheral nerve stimulator—this is useful in assessing degree of blockade, avoiding overdosage, and evaluating recovery

Use only **after** unconsciousness is produced and adequate general anesthesia is applied

Allow patients to recover from succinylcholine before use

Contraindicated with known hypersensitivity

(continued below)

Indications

Induction of skeletal muscle relaxation following the application of general anesthesia

Enhance pulmonary compliance during mechanical ventilation

Facilitate endotracheal intubation and prevent laryngospasm, especially when succinylcholine is contraindicated

Management of assisted respiration in status asthmaticus when conventional measures have failed

Pharmacokinetics

Onset of Action. Within 2–3 minutes

Peak Effects. 3–6 minutes

Duration of Action. Approximately 35–45 minutes

Tissue (Elimination) Half-Life. 89–161 minutes

There is a direct dose-dependent relationship influencing onset and duration of action. Hepatic and renal dysfunction may prolong elimination half-life

Metabolism. Primarily excreted unchanged in urine with minimal hepatic metabolism. Highly protein bound

Use with caution in hepatic or biliary dysfunction, obese patients, those with neuromuscular disease (especially myasthenia gravis), renal and heart failure, electrolyte abnormalities, pulmonary dysfunction, preexisting tachycardia, severe muscle spasm, history of hyperthermia, fractures, geriatric or debilitated individuals, and those on digitalis preparations

Overdosage may manifest as prolonged skeletal muscle weakness, decreased respiratory reserve with low tidal volume, and apnea. Manage by maintaining a patent airway and assisted ventilation until complete recovery is ensured. Excessive relaxation may be reversed by cholinesterase inhibitors such as pyridostigmine bromide (10–20 mg slow IV bolus) or neostigmine methylsulfate (0.5–2.5 mg slow IV bolus). Employ 0.6–1.2 mg atropine with or immediately before these agents to block adverse muscarinic effects. There is no established role for dialysis

Pancuronium Bromide (Pavulon)

Dosing Information

Initial Dose. 0.04–0.06 mg/kg IV bolus

Usual Dose Range. 0.06–0.1 mg/kg IV bolus

Maximum Dose. 0.16 mg/kg IV bolus

Titration Guideline

Suggested Regimen. Administer 0.01–0.015 mg/kg IV bolus every 25–60 minutes as necessary

How Supplied

1 mg/mL—10-mL vials of 10 mg

2 mg/mL—2-mL vials and syringes of 4 mg
5-mL vials and syringes of 10 mg

Potential Drug Interactions

Potentiation of Pancuronium Effects. Inhalation anesthetics, succinylcholine and other neuromuscular blocking agents, aminoglycosides, tetracycline, polymyxin, clindamycin, lincomycin, bacitracin, narcotic agonists, quinidine, quinine, magnesium sulfate, beta-blockers, high-dose lidocaine, diuretics, carbonic anhydrase inhibitors, amphotericin B, corticosteroids, tricyclic antidepressants in combination with halothane

Antagonism of Pancuronium Effects. Acetylcholine, theophylline, anticholinesterases, azathioprine, potassium, IV calcium

Principal Adverse Effects

CNS. Excessively prolonged neuromuscular blockade/skeletal muscle relaxation, malignant hyperthermia, flushing

Pulmonary. Apnea, wheezing, bronchospasm

CV. Tachycardia, hypertension, hypotension

GI. Salivation

Dermatological. Transient rash, sweating

Pancuronium Bromide (Pavulon) 50 mg in 250 mL

■ **Infusion Rate in mL/hr (pump setting)** ■ **Drug Dose in mg/hr**

mL/hr	mg/hr	mL/hr	mg/hr	mL/hr	mg/hr	mL/hr	mg/hr	mL/hr	mg/hr	mL/hr	mg/hr
1	0.2	21	4.2	41	8.2	61	12.2	81	16.2	101	20.2
2	0.4	22	4.4	42	8.4	62	12.4	82	16.4	102	20.4
3	0.6	23	4.6	43	8.6	63	12.6	83	16.6	103	20.6
4	0.8	24	4.8	44	8.8	64	12.8	84	16.8	104	20.8
5	1.0	25	5.0	45	9.0	65	13.0	85	17.0	105	21.0
6	1.2	26	5.2	46	9.2	66	13.2	86	17.2	106	21.2
7	1.4	27	5.4	47	9.4	67	13.4	87	17.4	107	21.4
8	1.6	28	5.6	48	9.6	68	13.6	88	17.6	108	21.6
9	1.8	29	5.8	49	9.8	69	13.8	89	17.8	109	21.8
10	2.0	30	6.0	50	10.0	70	14.0	90	18.0	110	22.0
11	2.2	31	6.2	51	10.2	71	14.2	91	18.2	111	22.2
12	2.4	32	6.4	52	10.4	72	14.4	92	18.4	112	22.4
13	2.6	33	6.6	53	10.6	73	14.6	93	18.6	113	22.6
14	2.8	34	6.8	54	10.8	74	14.8	94	18.8	114	22.8
15	3.0	35	7.0	55	11.0	75	15.0	95	19.0	115	23.0
16	3.2	36	7.2	56	11.2	76	15.2	96	19.2	116	23.2
17	3.4	37	7.4	57	11.4	77	15.4	97	19.4	117	23.4
18	3.6	38	7.6	58	11.6	78	15.6	98	19.6	118	23.6
19	3.8	39	7.8	59	11.8	79	15.8	99	19.8	119	23.8
20	4.0	40	8.0	60	12.0	80	16.0	100	20.0	120	24.0

DRUG DOSE in mg/kg/hr

Patient's Weight; rows: Infusion Rate in mL/hr

Infusion Rate in mL/hr \ kg (lbs)	40 (88)	45 (99)	50 (110)	55 (121)	60 (132)	65 (143)	70 (154)	75 (165)	80 (176)	85 (187)	90 (198)	95 (209)	100 (220)	105 (231)	110 (242)
5	0.03	0.02	0.02	0.02	0.02	0.02	0.01	0.01	0.01	0.01	0.01	0.01	0.01	0.01	0.01
10	0.05	0.04	0.04	0.04	0.03	0.03	0.03	0.03	0.03	0.02	0.02	0.02	0.02	0.02	0.02
15	0.08	0.07	0.06	0.05	0.05	0.05	0.04	0.04	0.04	0.04	0.03	0.03	0.03	0.03	0.03
20	0.10	0.09	0.08	0.07	0.07	0.06	0.06	0.05	0.05	0.05	0.04	0.04	0.04	0.04	0.04
25	0.13	0.11	0.10	0.09	0.08	0.08	0.07	0.07	0.06	0.06	0.06	0.05	0.05	0.05	0.05
30	0.15	0.13	0.12	0.11	0.10	0.09	0.09	0.08	0.08	0.07	0.07	0.06	0.06	0.06	0.05
35	0.17	0.16	0.14	0.13	0.12	0.11	0.10	0.09	0.09	0.08	0.08	0.07	0.07	0.07	0.06
40	0.20	0.18	0.16	0.15	0.13	0.12	0.11	0.11	0.10	0.09	0.09	0.08	0.08	0.08	0.07
45	0.22	0.20	0.18	0.16	0.15	0.14	0.13	0.12	0.11	0.11	0.10	0.09	0.09	0.09	0.08
50	0.25	0.22	0.20	0.18	0.17	0.15	0.14	0.13	0.13	0.12	0.11	0.11	0.10	0.10	0.09
55	0.28	0.24	0.22	0.20	0.18	0.17	0.16	0.15	0.14	0.13	0.12	0.12	0.11	0.10	0.10
60	0.30	0.27	0.24	0.22	0.20	0.18	0.17	0.16	0.15	0.14	0.13	0.13	0.12	0.11	0.11
65	0.32	0.29	0.26	0.24	0.22	0.20	0.19	0.17	0.16	0.15	0.14	0.14	0.13	0.12	0.12
70	0.35	0.31	0.28	0.25	0.23	0.22	0.20	0.19	0.17	0.16	0.16	0.15	0.14	0.13	0.13
75	0.38	0.33	0.30	0.27	0.25	0.23	0.21	0.20	0.19	0.18	0.17	0.16	0.15	0.14	0.14
80	0.40	0.36	0.32	0.29	0.27	0.25	0.23	0.21	0.20	0.19	0.18	0.17	0.16	0.15	0.15
85	0.43	0.38	0.34	0.31	0.28	0.26	0.24	0.23	0.21	0.20	0.19	0.18	0.17	0.16	0.15
90	0.45	0.40	0.36	0.33	0.30	0.28	0.26	0.24	0.22	0.21	0.20	0.19	0.18	0.17	0.16
95	0.47	0.42	0.38	0.35	0.32	0.29	0.27	0.25	0.24	0.22	0.21	0.20	0.19	0.18	0.17
100	0.50	0.44	0.40	0.36	0.33	0.31	0.29	0.27	0.25	0.24	0.22	0.21	0.20	0.19	0.18
105	0.52	0.47	0.42	0.38	0.35	0.32	0.30	0.28	0.26	0.25	0.23	0.22	0.21	0.20	0.19
110	0.55	0.49	0.44	0.40	0.37	0.34	0.31	0.29	0.28	0.26	0.24	0.23	0.22	0.21	0.20
115	0.57	0.51	0.46	0.42	0.38	0.35	0.33	0.31	0.29	0.27	0.26	0.24	0.23	0.22	0.21
120	0.60	0.53	0.48	0.44	0.40	0.37	0.34	0.32	0.30	0.28	0.27	0.25	0.24	0.23	0.22

Phenobarbital Sodium (Luminal)

Pharmacology

Nonselective CNS depressant of the barbiturate class

Produces drowsiness, sedation, hypnosis, and anticonvulsant effects by depressing the sensory cortex, motor activity, and cerebellar function

Raises seizure threshold of motor cortex and limits spread of seizure activity by reducing monosynaptic and polysynaptic transmission, thereby causing decreased neuroexcitability

Produces respiratory depression and may reduce blood pressure and heart rate

Reduces REM phase and stages III and IV of sleep

No significant analgesic effect at subanesthetic doses

Administrative Guidelines

Administer infusion via precision control device

Monitor ECG, vital signs, and serum drug levels

Determine complete blood counts, hepatic and renal chemistries before and intermittently during long-term therapy

Administer via large vein or, if possible, central line

Restrict IV use to emergency seizure states or situations in which other routes of administration are not feasible, or prompt action is required

Never administer faster than 60 mg/min—more rapid delivery may produce respiratory depression, apnea, laryngospasm, and hypotension

Tolerance, psychological dependence, and physical dependence may develop with prolonged use

Parenteral solutions are highly alkaline. Subcutaneous injections may result in local reactions, including tissue necrosis. Apply moist heat and 0.5% procaine injection into affected area if extravasation occurs

(continued below)

Indications

Sedation and hypnosis for short-term insomnia

Management of partial and grand mal (tonic-clonic) seizures usually in conjunction with phenytoin or other anticonvulsive agents

Termination of seizure recurrence after initial cessation with other anticonvulsants

Management of status epilepticus unresponsive to conventional therapy

Preanesthetic agent

Pharmacokinetics

Onset of Action. Within 5 minutes

Peak Effects. Within 30 minutes

Duration of Action. Usually 4–6 hours but may last up to 10 hours

Plasma Half-Life. 2–6 days

Metabolism. Via hepatic microsomal enzymes with 20–50% eliminated unchanged in urine

Intra-arterial injection may result in gangrene. Suggested treatment involves release of tourniquet or restrictive apparel, injection of 10 mL of 1.0% procaine solution into the artery to relieve spasm, anticoagulant therapy to prevent thrombosis, supportive therapy, and possible brachioplexus block

Discontinue administration if patient experiences pain or adverse dermatologic response is noted—skin lesions may precede potentially fatal reactions

Minimize dose when managing convulsions because at least 15 minutes is required for peak CNS effects. Continued administration before seizure control may produce excessive brain concentrations and barbiturate-induced depression

Reduce dose in elderly or debilitated patients and those with renal or hepatic disease

Contraindicated in those with known hypersensitivity, history of porphyria, severe hepatic or pulmonary dysfunction, or previous addiction to sedative hypnotic agents; and in nephritic patients requiring large doses

(continued on page 222)

Use cautiously in patients with acute or chronic pain, in elderly or debilitated patients, in patients with fever, severe anemia, hyperthyroidism, diabetes mellitus, shock, hypotension, hypertension, renal insufficiency, pulmonary disease, cardiovascular disease, hepatic disease, or hypoadrenal function; or in patients performing tasks requiring mental alertness or physical coordination

Overdosage may manifest by CNS and respiratory depression. Shock with multisystem organ failure may ensue. A "flat" electroencephalogram may be seen but should not be construed as clinical death. Treatment includes supportive measures, alkalinization of the urine to facilitate renal excretion, and rolling the patient from side to side every 30 minutes. Hemodialysis may be employed if shock or anuria is present

Dosing Information

IV Bolus Dose for Daytime Sedation. 30–120 mg daily in 2–3 divided doses

IV Bolus Dose for Bedtime Hypnosis. 100–320 mg IV

Subsequent Dosing. After 5 minutes, if clinical response is inadequate, administer small doses slowly until desired effect

Initial IV Bolus Dose for Acute Convulsions. 20–600 mg over 5–10 minutes

Subsequent Dosing. After 6 hours may administer 200–300 mg over 5–6 minutes. Repeat every 6 hours as necessary

Maximum IV Dose. 20 mg/kg

Do not administer IV bolus faster than 60 mg/min

Therapeutic Levels

10–25 μg/mL

Potential Drug Interactions

Potentiation of Phenobarbital Effects. Alcohol, CNS depressants, monoamine oxidase inhibitors, disulfiram, valproic acid

Possibly Antagonized by Phenobarbital. Digitoxin, oral anticoagulants such as warfarin, corticosteroids, griseofulvin, phenytoin, doxycycline, oral contraceptives, estrogen, theophylline, rifampin, beta-blockers, quinidine, acetaminophen

Possibly Potentiated by Phenobarbital. Furosemide and phenytoin

Phenobarbital Sodium (Luminal)

How Supplied

30 mg/mL—1-mL syringe (Tubex) of 30 mg

60 mg/mL—1-mL syringe (Tubex) of 60 mg

65 mg/mL—1-mL vial of 65 mg

130 mg/mL—ampuls, vials, and syringes of 1 mL (130 mg)

Principal Adverse Effects

CNS. Drowsiness, CNS depression, dizziness, insomnia, anxiety, lethargy, confusion, agitation, residual sedation, hallucinations, vertigo, ataxia, delirium, hyperkinesia

Pulmonary. Respiratory depression, hypoventilation, apnea, bronchospasm, and cough

CV. Circulatory collapse, hypotension, bradycardia, syncope

GI. Nausea, vomiting, diarrhea, constipation, epigastric pain, liver damage with long-term use

Heme. Megaloblastic anemia, thrombocytopenic purpura, leukopenia

Dermatological. Rash, exfoliative dermatitis, Stevens-Johnson syndrome, pain at injection site

Allergic. Serum sickness, urticaria, angioneurotic edema

Miscellaneous. Pain syndrome of myalgia, neuralgia, or arthralgia and thrombophlebitis

Phenylephrine Hydrochloride (Neo-Synephrine)

Pharmacology

Sympathomimetic amine that acts predominantly on postsynaptic alpha-adrenergic receptors

Alpha-adrenergic effects are believed to be mediated by inhibiting adenyl cyclase activity and cyclic adenosine monophosphate formation

No significant beta-adrenergic effects with therapeutic doses. May stimulate beta$_1$-receptors and adenyl cyclase at high doses

May indirectly release norepinephrine from storage sites

Potent vasoconstrictor of resistance vessels, which raises blood pressure—venous capacitance vessels are less affected but may result in decreased venous return

Constricts pulmonary blood vessels and increases pulmonary artery pressure and resistance

Constricts coronary blood vessels but usually augments coronary blood flow

(continued below)

Administration Guidelines

Administer infusion via precision control device

Monitor ECG and blood pressure continuously; carefully follow vital signs, acid-base status, and hemodynamic variables

Correct any underlying hypovolemia, if possible, before use; do **not** use as sole treatment in hypovolemic patients

Electrolytes, hypoxia, and acidosis should be reversed before and during phenylephrine therapy

Do not admix with oxidizing agents, metals, or ferric salts

Administer via central line, if possible, or large vein (antecubital site recommended)

Carefully observe infusion site for free-flow, blanching, and extravasation

Extravasation requires immediate discontinuation of infusion and subcutaneous infiltration of 5–10 mg phentolamine in 10–15 mL saline

(continued below)

Constricts cerebral and renal vessels but preserves blood flow to these organs

May reduce renal, skeletal muscle, mesenteric, and skin blood supply

Myocardial oxygen requirements are usually increased and tachydysrhythmias are occasionally seen, especially after spinal anesthesia

Reflex bradycardia (vagally mediated) commonly occurs secondary to increased arterial blood pressure; this response can be blocked by atropine

No significant spinal cord or CNS stimulation at usual doses

Contraindicated in those with known hypersensitivity (contains sodium metabisulfite), severe hypertension, ventricular tachycardia, or peripheral or mesenteric ischemia

Use with caution in patients with severe arteriosclerosis, heart block, bradycardia, hyperthyroidism, myocardial infarction, cardiovascular disease, hepatitis, pancreatitis, and the elderly

Overdosage may manifest as severe hypoperfusion with acidosis, diffuse vasoconstriction, hypertension, headache, seizures, palpitations, dysrhythmias, and paresthesias. Manage with supportive measures and alpha-adrenergic blockade with phentolamine IV. There is no established role for dialysis

Phenylephrine Hydrochloride (Neo-Synephrine)

Indications

Short-term support of blood pressure in drug-induced hypotension or hypersensitivity reactions and nonhypovolemic shock (especially low-resistance shock)

Control of paroxysmal supraventricular tachycardia

Prolongation of spinal anesthesia, vasoconstriction in regional anesthesia, and maintenance of blood pressure during inhalational and spinal anesthesia

Pharmacokinetics

Onset of Action. Almost immediately

Peak Effects. Within 15 minutes

Duration of Action. 15–20 minutes

Metabolism. Via liver and intestine but metabolites and route of elimination not established

Dosing Information

IV Bolus Dose. 100–500 μg over 1 minute. Repeat every 10–15 minutes as necessary

Initial Infusion Rate. 100–180 μg/min

Maintenance Infusion Range. 40–60 μg/min

Maximum Infusion Rate. Not specified by manufacturer

Titration Guideline

Suggested Regimen. Adjust infusion by 10–100 μg/min every 10–15 minutes as required to obtain desired blood pressure

How Supplied

10 mg/mL—1-mL ampuls of 10 mg

Potential Drug Interactions

Potentiation of Phenylephrine Effects. Halogenated hydrocarbon anesthetics, oxytocic agents, monoamine oxidase inhibitors, tricyclic antidepressants, bretylium, ergot alkaloids, guanethidine, sympathomimetics, atropine

Antagonism of Phenylephrine Effects. Alpha-adrenergic blockers, phenothiazines, beta-blockers, tricyclic antidepressants

Possible Potentiation of Dysrhythmias When Phenylephrine Is Used Concomitantly. Digitalis glycosides, guanethidine, sympathomimetics, bretylium, reserpine, halogenated hydrocarbon anesthetics

Phenylephrine Hydrochloride (Neo-Synephrine)

Principal Adverse Effects

CNS. Anxiety, headache, excitability, restlessness, weakness, dizziness, seizures, cerebral hemorrhage, and paresthesias

Pulmonary. Respiratory distress

CV. Chest pain, reduced cardiac output, bradycardia, cardiac dysrhythmias, hypertension, hypotension, peripheral and visceral vasoconstriction

GI. Vomiting

Dermatological. Sloughing and necrosis of skin at infusion site, blanching or skin pallor

Phenylephrine Hydrochloride (Neo-Synephrine) 50 mg in 500 mL

■ Infusion Rate in mL/hr (pump setting) ■ Drug Dose in µg/min

mL/hr	µg/min	mL/hr	µg/min	mL/hr	µg/min	mL/hr	µg/min	mL/hr	µg/min	mL/hr	µg/min
1	1.7	21	35.0	41	68.3	61	101.7	81	135.0	101	168.3
2	3.3	22	36.7	42	70.0	62	103.3	82	136.7	102	170.0
3	5.0	23	38.3	43	71.7	63	105.0	83	138.3	103	171.7
4	6.7	24	40.0	44	73.3	64	106.7	84	140.0	104	173.3
5	8.3	25	41.7	45	75.0	65	108.3	85	141.7	105	175.0
6	10.0	26	43.3	46	76.7	66	110.0	86	143.3	106	176.7
7	11.7	27	45.0	47	78.3	67	111.7	87	145.0	107	178.3
8	13.3	28	46.7	48	80.0	68	113.3	88	146.7	108	180.0
9	15.0	29	48.3	49	81.7	69	115.0	89	148.3	109	181.7
10	16.7	30	50.0	50	83.3	70	116.7	90	150.0	110	183.3
11	18.3	31	51.7	51	85.0	71	118.3	91	151.7	111	185.0
12	20.0	32	53.3	52	86.7	72	120.0	92	153.3	112	186.7
13	21.7	33	55.0	53	88.3	73	121.7	93	155.0	113	188.3
14	23.3	34	56.7	54	90.0	74	123.3	94	156.7	114	190.0
15	25.0	35	58.3	55	91.7	75	125.0	95	158.3	115	191.7
16	26.7	36	60.0	56	93.3	76	126.7	96	160.0	116	193.3
17	28.3	37	61.7	57	95.0	77	128.3	97	161.7	117	195.0
18	30.0	38	63.3	58	96.7	78	130.0	98	163.3	118	196.7
19	31.7	39	65.0	59	98.3	79	131.7	99	165.0	119	198.3
20	33.3	40	66.7	60	100.0	80	133.3	100	166.7	120	200.0

Infusion Rate in mL/hr (pump setting)	Drug Dose in mg/min	Infusion Rate in mL/hr (pump setting)	Drug Dose in mg/min	Infusion Rate in mL/hr (pump setting)	Drug Dose in mg/min	Infusion Rate in mL/hr (pump setting)	Drug Dose in mg/min	Infusion Rate in mL/hr (pump setting)	Drug Dose in mg/min	Infusion Rate in mL/hr (pump setting)	Drug Dose in mg/min
1	3.3	21	70.0	41	136.7	61	203.3	81	270.0	101	336.7
2	6.7	22	73.3	42	140.0	62	206.7	82	273.3	102	340.0
3	10.0	23	76.7	43	143.3	63	210.0	83	276.7	103	343.3
4	13.3	24	80.0	44	146.7	64	213.3	84	280.0	104	346.7
5	16.7	25	83.3	45	150.0	65	216.7	85	283.3	105	350.0
6	20.0	26	86.7	46	153.3	66	220.0	86	286.7	106	353.3
7	23.3	27	90.0	47	156.7	67	223.3	87	290.0	107	356.7
8	26.7	28	93.3	48	160.0	68	226.7	88	293.3	108	360.0
9	30.0	29	96.7	49	163.3	69	230.0	89	296.7	109	363.3
10	33.3	30	100.0	50	166.7	70	233.3	90	300.0	110	366.7
11	36.7	31	103.3	51	170.0	71	236.7	91	303.3	111	370.0
12	40.0	32	106.7	52	173.3	72	240.0	92	306.7	112	373.3
13	43.3	33	110.0	53	176.7	73	243.3	93	310.0	113	376.7
14	46.7	34	113.3	54	180.0	74	246.7	94	313.3	114	380.0
15	50.0	35	116.7	55	183.3	75	250.0	95	316.7	115	383.3
16	53.3	36	120.0	56	186.7	76	253.3	96	320.0	116	386.7
17	56.7	37	123.3	57	190.0	77	256.7	97	323.3	117	390.0
18	60.0	38	126.7	58	193.3	78	260.0	98	326.7	118	393.3
19	63.3	39	130.0	59	196.7	79	263.3	99	330.0	119	396.7
20	66.7	40	133.3	60	200.0	80	266.7	100	333.3	120	400.0

Procainamide Hydrochloride (Pronestyl)

Pharmacology

Vaughn-Williams class 1A antiarrhythmic agent with local anesthetic and anticholinergic properties

Stabilizes cell membranes by interacting with fast sodium channels in a time-dependent and voltage-dependent manner

Electrophysiologic effects include suppressing His-Purkinje and ectopic pacemaker automaticity; decreasing conduction velocity and excitability of atria, ventricles, and His-Purkinje system; prolonging refractory period and action potential duration in atria, ventricles, and His-Purkinje network; shortening atrioventricular node effective refractory period and accelerating atrioventricular conduction (vagolytic effect); no significant sinoatrial node effects but may slightly increase heart rate

Prolongs P-R and QT intervals on the ECG but no major QRS lengthening at therapeutic doses

May directly depress myocardial contractility, reduce blood pressure by peripheral vasodilation, and lower pulmonary artery pressure

Administrative Guidelines

Administer infusion via precision control device

Monitor blood pressure continuously during IV loading and place patient in supine position—temporarily discontinue if greater than 15-mmHg drop in systolic pressure noted

Continuously follow the ECG—prolongation of the P-R interval, proarrhythmic responses, and excessive prolongation of QRS (>50%) or QT intervals indicate myocardial toxicity; discontinue infusion and consider alternative treatment

Carefully follow electrolytes, magnesium, calcium, vital signs, and acid-base status

Determine complete blood count before therapy and weekly during therapy. The appearance of infection, bruising, or bleeding may reflect bone marrow toxicity and mandates a complete blood count measurement. Discontinue procainamide if hematologic abnormalities are identified

(continued below)

Indications

Prophylaxis and treatment of life-threatening and symptomatic ventricular dysrhythmias

Treatment of wide complex tachycardias of uncertain origin

Unlabeled Uses. Asymptomatic ventricular dysrhythmias; conversion of atrial fibrillation and flutter to sinus rhythm; maintenance of sinus rhythm following conversion of atrial flutter or fibrillation; atrial premature complexes; paroxysmal atrial and junctional tachycardias; malignant hyperthermia

Except for life-threatening ventricular dysrhythmias, there is no definitive evidence that procainamide has a beneficial effect on mortality or sudden death

A positive antinuclear antibody may develop in the absence of symptoms of lupus erythematosus (about 50% of patients). Continuation of treatment is appropriate if clinically warranted or until lupus symptoms develop

Always dilute before use—recommended 5% dextrose injection USP

Slight yellow discoloration is normal—discard solution if darker than amber color observed

Periodic drug levels are recommended, especially with renal or hepatic dysfunction, if toxicity is suspected, or if there is lack of efficacy

Reduced doses are required with renal or congestive heart failure and during amiodarone therapy—follow serum NAPA and procainamide levels

Cardioversion or slow atrioventricular conduction before procainamide therapy in patients with atrial fibrillation or flutter associated with a rapid ven[illegible]icular response

Contraindicated in patients with known h[illegible] sensitivity (may contain sodium metabis[illegible]

Procainamide Hydrochloride (Pronestyl)

Procainamide Hydrochloride (Pronestyl)

Pharmacokinetics

Onset of Action. Almost immediately

Peak Effects. Approximately 5–15 minutes

Duration of Action. Variable owing to hepatic acetylation (at least 1–2 hours)

IV Bolus (Distribution) Half-Life. Approximately 12–18 minutes

IV Infusion (Elimination) Half-Life. 2.5–4.7 hours

Metabolism. Via acetylation in liver to N-acetylprocainamide (NAPA), which is metabolically active with a half-life of 7 hours in patients with normal renal function. 40–70% of procainamide excreted unchanged in urine

de pointes, second-degree and third-degree heart block without a functioning artificial ventricular pacemaker, systemic lupus erythematosus, and myasthenia gravis (may increase muscle weakness)

Use with caution if baseline QT interval prolonged; with rapid atrial fibrillation (may accelerate the ventricular response); in patients taking digitalis glycosides; in patients with heart block or conduction disturbances, renal or hepatic disease, congestive heart failure, preexisting cytopenias or bone marrow depression, or ventricular dysrhythmias with severe underlying organic heart disease; in asymptomatic nonsustained ventricular dysrhythmias; and concurrently with other 1A antiarrhythmic drugs

Overdosage may manifest with new dysrhythmias; conduction abnormalities; excessive prolongation of P-R, QRS, and QT intervals; hypotension; tremor; and CNS and respiratory depression. Provide supportive measures because there is no specific antidote. Infusion of $\frac{1}{8}$ molar sodium lactate injection has reportedly lessened the cardiotoxic effects. Hemodialysis removes procainamide and NAPA, but peritoneal dialysis is ineffective

Dosing Information

IV Loading Dose. 20–30 mg/min procainamide diluted in 5% dextrose injection USP up to 600 mg total dose. Thereafter, wait 10 minutes for equilibration before administering additional drug

Maximum IV Loading Dose. 1000 mg

Maintenance Infusion Range. 2–6 mg/min

Maximum Infusion Rate. 6 mg/min

Titration Guideline

Suggested Regimen. Adjust infusion by 1 mg/min and consider additional 20–30 mg/min IV bolus dosing as required for dysrhythmia control

Therapeutic Serum Levels

Procainamide. 4–10 μg/mL

NAPA. 10–30 μg/mL

Dysrhythmia control may correlate best with procainamide level

Potential Drug Interactions

Potentiation of Procainamide Effects. Beta-blockers, quinidine, trimethoprim, cimetidine, ranitidine, hypotensive agents, phenytoin, amiodarone, anticholinergic drugs

Possibly Potentiated by Procainamide. Lidocaine, succinylcholine and other neuromuscular blocking agents, quinidine, disopyramide, phenytoin, propranolol

Possibly Suppressed by Procainamide. Digitalis toxicity

Procainamide Hydrochloride (Pronestyl)

How Supplied

100 mg/mL—10-mL vials of 1000 mg

500 mg/mL—2-mL vials and syringes of 1000 mg
4-mL syringes of 2000 mg

Principal Adverse Effects

CNS. Weakness, psychosis, hallucinations, depression, altered consciousness, seizures, proximal myopathy, and giddiness

CV. Hypotension, serious proarrhythmic responses including ventricular tachycardia and fibrillation, atrioventricular block, acceleration of ventricular rate in atrial fibrillation or flutter, asystole, arterial embolization following conversion of atrial fibrillation or flutter to sinus rhythm

GI. Nausea, vomiting, abdominal pain, diarrhea, anorexia, hepatic dysfunction, bitter taste

Heme. Agranulocytosis, thrombocytopenia, neutropenia, hemolytic anemia, red cell aplasia, eosinophilia

Dermatological. Vasculitis, flushing, pruritus, rash

Allergic. Lupuslike syndrome, fever, chills, urticaria, angioneurotic edema

Miscellaneous. Hypergammaglobulinemia, Sjögren's syndrome

Procainamide Hydrochloride (Pronestyl) 2 g in 500 mL

Infusion Rate in mL/hr (pump setting)	Drug Dose in mg/min	Infusion Rate in mL/hr (pump setting)	Drug Dose in mg/min	Infusion Rate in mL/hr (pump setting)	Drug Dose in mg/min	Infusion Rate in mL/hr (pump setting)	Drug Dose in mg/min	Infusion Rate in mL/hr (pump setting)	Drug Dose in mg/min	Infusion Rate in mL/hr (pump setting)	Drug Dose in mg/min
1	0.07	21	1.40	41	2.73	61	4.07	81	5.40	101	6.73
2	0.13	22	1.47	42	2.80	62	4.13	82	5.47	102	6.80
3	0.20	23	1.53	43	2.87	63	4.20	83	5.53	103	6.87
4	0.27	24	1.60	44	2.93	64	4.27	84	5.60	104	6.93
5	0.33	25	1.67	45	3.00	65	4.33	85	5.67	105	7.00
6	0.40	26	1.73	46	3.07	66	4.40	86	5.73	106	7.07
7	0.47	27	1.80	47	3.13	67	4.47	87	5.80	107	7.13
8	0.53	28	1.87	48	3.20	68	4.53	88	5.87	108	7.20
9	0.60	29	1.93	49	3.27	69	4.60	89	5.93	109	7.27
10	0.67	30	2.00	50	3.33	70	4.67	90	6.00	110	7.33
11	0.73	31	2.07	51	3.40	71	4.73	91	6.07	111	7.40
12	0.80	32	2.13	52	3.47	72	4.80	92	6.13	112	7.47
13	0.87	33	2.20	53	3.53	73	4.87	93	6.20	113	7.53
14	0.93	34	2.27	54	3.60	74	4.93	94	6.27	114	7.60
15	1.00	35	2.33	55	3.67	75	5.00	95	6.33	115	7.67
16	1.07	36	2.40	56	3.73	76	5.07	96	6.40	116	7.73
17	1.13	37	2.47	57	3.80	77	5.13	97	6.47	117	7.80
18	1.20	38	2.53	58	3.87	78	5.20	98	6.53	118	7.87
19	1.27	39	2.60	59	3.93	79	5.27	99	6.60	119	7.93
20	1.33	40	2.67	60	4.00	80	5.33	100	6.67	120	8.00

Procainamide Hydrochloride (Pronestyl) 4 g in 500 mL

Infusion Rate in mL/hr (pump setting)	Drug Dose in mg/min	Infusion Rate in mL/hr (pump setting)	Drug Dose in mg/min	Infusion Rate in mL/hr (pump setting)	Drug Dose in mg/min	Infusion Rate in mL/hr (pump setting)	Drug Dose in mg/min	Infusion Rate in mL/hr (pump setting)	Drug Dose in mg/min	Infusion Rate in mL/hr (pump setting)	Drug Dose in mg/min
1	0.13	21	2.80	41	5.47	61	8.13	81	10.80	101	13.47
2	0.27	22	2.93	42	5.60	62	8.27	82	10.93	102	13.60
3	0.40	23	3.07	43	5.73	63	8.40	83	11.07	103	13.73
4	0.53	24	3.20	44	5.87	64	8.53	84	11.20	104	13.87
5	0.67	25	3.33	45	6.00	65	8.67	85	11.33	105	14.00
6	0.80	26	3.47	46	6.13	66	8.80	86	11.47	106	14.13
7	0.93	27	3.60	47	6.27	67	8.93	87	11.60	107	14.27
8	1.07	28	3.73	48	6.40	68	9.07	88	11.73	108	14.40
9	1.20	29	3.87	49	6.53	69	9.20	89	11.87	109	14.53
10	1.33	30	4.00	50	6.67	70	9.33	90	12.00	110	14.67
11	1.47	31	4.13	51	6.80	71	9.47	91	12.13	111	14.80
12	1.60	32	4.27	52	6.93	72	9.60	92	12.27	112	14.93
13	1.73	33	4.40	53	7.07	73	9.73	93	12.40	113	15.07
14	1.87	34	4.53	54	7.20	74	9.87	94	12.53	114	15.20
15	2.00	35	4.67	55	7.33	75	10.00	95	12.67	115	15.33
16	2.13	36	4.80	56	7.47	76	10.13	96	12.80	116	15.47
17	2.27	37	4.93	57	7.60	77	10.27	97	12.93	117	15.60
18	2.40	38	5.07	58	7.73	78	10.40	98	13.07	118	15.73
19	2.53	39	5.20	59	7.87	79	10.53	99	13.20	119	15.87
20	2.67	40	5.33	60	8.00	80	10.67	100	13.33	120	16.00

Propranolol Hydrochloride (Inderal)

Pharmacology

Competitive and nonselective beta-adrenergic blocking agent

Principal effects on myocardial ($beta_1$) and bronchial plus vascular smooth muscle ($beta_2$) receptors

Highly lipid soluble—no intrinsic sympathomimetic activity

Important membrane stabilizing/anesthetic action

Usually decreases myocardial oxygen consumption by reducing heart rate, blood pressure, and cardiac contractility

Decreases myocardial automaticity and sinoatrial and atrioventricular node activity

May block renin release and reduce platelet aggregation, portal pressure, hepatic and renal blood flow, and glomerular filtration rate

Inhibits glycogenolysis, free fatty acid and insulin release, and red blood cell affinity for oxygen via 2,3-diphosphoglyceric acid

Administrative Guidelines

Carefully monitor ECG and blood pressure

Avoid abrupt discontinuation of long-term therapy in patients with ischemic heart disease

Propranolol may elevate serum transaminase and blood urea nitrogen

Contraindicated in those with known hypersensitivity, cardiogenic shock, bronchial asthma, hypertensive crisis, sinus bradycardia, second-degree or third-degree atrioventricular block. Raynaud's syndrome, and possibly myasthenia gravis

Use with caution in patients with glaucoma, Wolff-Parkinson-White syndrome, thyrotoxicosis, renal or hepatic dysfunction, nonallergic bronchospasm, diabetes; before major surgery; with sinus node dysfunction; or during use of myocardial depressant anesthetics

Overdosage requires supportive measures—induce emesis or perform gastric lavage. Atropine, isoproterenol, or 5–10 mg IV glucagon may be beneficial to antagonize beta-blockade. Dialysis is not useful

Indications

Control of stable and unstable angina

Reduction of cardiovascular morbidity and mortality after myocardial infarction

Management of hypertension

Prophylaxis and therapy of supraventricular and ventricular dysrhythmias

Adjunctive treatment of pheochromocytoma and symptomatic or malignant dysrhythmias of thyrotoxicosis

Control of benign and familial essential tremor

Therapy of idiopathic hypertrophic subaortic stenosis

Unlabeled Uses. Reduction of portal pressure in cirrhotic gastrointestinal bleeding; diastolic heart failure; schizophrenia; acute panic disorders

Propranolol Hydrochloride (Inderal)

Pharmacokinetics

Onset of Action. Almost immediately

Peak Effects. Within 1 minute

Duration of Action. Approximately 5 minutes after single IV bolus

IV Bolus Distribution Half-Life. 10 minutes

IV Bolus Elimination Half-Life. 2.3 hours

Dosing Information

Initial IV Bolus Dose. 0.5–3 mg slow IV push—do not exceed 1 mg/min

May repeat above dose after 2 minutes; thereafter, administer further doses at intervals of 4 hours

Initial Infusion Rate. 1 mg/hr

Maintenance Infusion Range. 2–3 mg/hr

Maximum Infusion Rate. 3 mg/hr

Intravenous use **only** for life-threatening dysrhythmias or dysrhythmias during anesthesia and in the immediate postoperative setting

Titration Guideline

Suggested Regimen. Adjust infusion by 0.5–0.1 mg/hr as required

How Supplied

1 mg/mL—1-mL ampuls of 1 mg

Potential Drug Interactions

Potentiation of Propranolol Effects. Reserpine, angiotensin converting enzyme inhibitors, calcium channel blockers, chlorpromazine, cimetidine, oral contraceptives, furosemide, lidocaine, hydralazine, prazosin, clonidine, phenytoin (IV), quinidine, procainamide, high-dose ergot alkaloids

Antagonism of Propranolol Effects. Isoproterenol, dobutamine, dopamine, norepinephrine, phenobarbital, rifampin, thyroid hormone, smoking, indomethacin, salicylates, atropine, tricyclic antidepressants

Possibly Antagonized by Propranolol. Levodopa, theophylline

Possibly Potentiated by Propranolol. Succinylcholine, tubocurarine, digitalis, insulin

Propranolol Hydrochloride (Inderal)

Principal Adverse Effects

CNS. Mental status changes, depression, fatigue, vertigo, dizziness, catatonia, bizarre dreams, anxiety, tinnitus, headache, dysphonia, acute organic brain syndrome, emotional lability, visual disturbances, weakness, lightheadedness, ataxia, hearing loss, insomnia, impotence, ptosis, peripheral neuropathy, paresthesia, myotonia

Pulmonary. Bronchospasm, cough, wheezing, rhinitis

CV. Bradycardia, heart block, hypotension, congestive failure, syncope, chest pain, arterial insufficiency, palpitations, shock, cardiac arrest, edema, tachycardia, cerebrovascular accident

GI. Mesenteric insufficiency, nausea, vomiting, diarrhea, ischemic colitis, constipation, abdominal cramps, pancreatitis, hepatomegaly, retroperitoneal fibrosis, dry mouth, anorexia

GU. Impotence, nocturia, dysuria, Peyronie's disease

Heme. Agranulocytosis, purpura, thrombocytopenic purpura

(continued below)

Allergic. Rash, fever, pharyngitis, hypersensitivity reactions

Dermatological. Skin necrosis, psoriasiform rash, alopecia, pruritus, hyperhidrosis

Miscellaneous. Lupuslike syndrome, arthralgia, conjunctivitis, visual disturbances, eye irritation, hyperglycemia, and hypoglycemia

Propranolol Hydrochloride (Inderal) 15 mg in 500 mL

■ Infusion Rate in mL/hr (pump setting) ■ Drug Dose in mg/hr

mL/hr	mg/hr	mL/hr	mg/hr	mL/hr	mg/hr	mL/hr	mg/hr	mL/hr	mg/hr	mL/hr	mg/hr
1	0.03	21	0.63	41	1.23	61	1.83	81	2.43	101	3.03
2	0.06	22	0.66	42	1.26	62	1.86	82	2.46	102	3.06
3	0.09	23	0.69	43	1.29	63	1.89	83	2.49	103	3.09
4	0.12	24	0.72	44	1.32	64	1.92	84	2.52	104	3.12
5	0.15	25	0.75	45	1.35	65	1.95	85	2.55	105	3.15
6	0.18	26	0.78	46	1.38	66	1.98	86	2.58	106	3.18
7	0.21	27	0.81	47	1.41	67	2.01	87	2.61	107	3.21
8	0.24	28	0.84	48	1.44	68	2.04	88	2.64	108	3.24
9	0.27	29	0.87	49	1.47	69	2.07	89	2.67	109	3.27
10	0.30	30	0.90	50	1.50	70	2.10	90	2.70	110	3.30
11	0.33	31	0.93	51	1.53	71	2.13	91	2.73	111	3.33
12	0.36	32	0.96	52	1.56	72	2.16	92	2.76	112	3.36
13	0.39	33	0.99	53	1.59	73	2.19	93	2.79	113	3.39
14	0.42	34	1.02	54	1.62	74	2.22	94	2.82	114	3.42
15	0.45	35	1.05	55	1.65	75	2.25	95	2.85	115	3.45
16	0.48	36	1.08	56	1.68	76	2.28	96	2.88	116	3.48
17	0.51	37	1.11	57	1.71	77	2.31	97	2.91	117	4.51
18	0.54	38	1.14	58	1.74	78	2.34	98	2.94	118	3.54
19	0.57	39	1.17	59	1.77	79	2.37	99	2.97	119	3.57
20	0.60	40	1.20	60	1.80	80	2.40	100	3.00	120	3.60

Infusion Rate in mL/hr (pump setting)	Drug Dose in mg/hr	Infusion Rate in mL/hr (pump setting)	Drug Dose in mg/hr	Infusion Rate in mL/hr (pump setting)	Drug Dose in mg/hr	Infusion Rate in mL/hr (pump setting)	Drug Dose in mg/hr	Infusion Rate in mL/hr (pump setting)	Drug Dose in mg/hr	Infusion Rate in mL/hr (pump setting)	Drug Dose in mg/hr
1	0.06	21	1.26	41	2.46	61	3.66	81	4.86	101	6.06
2	0.12	22	1.32	42	2.52	62	3.72	82	4.92	102	6.12
3	0.18	23	1.38	43	2.58	63	3.78	83	4.98	103	6.18
4	0.24	24	1.44	44	2.64	64	3.84	84	5.04	104	6.24
5	0.30	25	1.50	45	2.70	65	3.90	85	5.10	105	6.30
6	0.36	26	1.56	46	2.76	66	3.96	86	5.16	106	6.36
7	0.42	27	1.62	47	2.82	67	4.02	87	5.22	107	6.42
8	0.48	28	1.68	48	2.88	68	4.08	88	5.28	108	6.48
9	0.54	29	1.74	49	2.94	69	4.14	89	5.34	109	6.54
10	0.60	30	1.80	50	3.00	70	4.20	90	5.40	110	6.60
11	0.66	31	1.86	51	3.06	71	4.26	91	5.46	111	6.66
12	0.72	32	1.92	52	3.12	72	4.32	92	5.52	112	6.72
13	0.78	33	1.98	53	3.18	73	4.38	93	5.58	113	6.78
14	0.84	34	2.04	54	3.24	74	4.44	94	5.64	114	6.84
15	0.90	35	2.10	55	3.30	75	4.50	95	5.70	115	6.90
16	0.96	36	2.16	56	3.36	76	4.56	96	5.76	116	6.96
17	1.02	37	2.22	57	3.42	77	4.62	97	5.82	117	7.02
18	1.08	38	2.28	58	3.48	78	4.68	98	5.88	118	7.08
19	1.14	39	2.34	59	3.54	79	4.74	99	5.94	119	7.14
20	1.20	40	2.40	60	3.60	80	4.80	100	6.00	120	7.20

Ranitidine Hydrochloride (Zantac)

Pharmacology

Reduces gastric acid secretion by competitive inhibition of histamine on H_2 receptors in parietal cells

Protects gastric mucosa from irritant effects of nonsteroidal anti-inflammatory agents

Indirectly reduces pepsin secretion

Causes bacterial overgrowth and delay in gastric emptying

May inhibit gastroesophageal reflux

Administrative Guidelines

Administer infusion via precision control device

After 5 days of IV therapy at daily doses of 400 mg, monitor daily serum ALT levels until infusion is discontinued

Contraindicated in patients with acute porphyria or known hypersensitivity

Use with caution in patients with hepatic or renal impairment and in nursing women

Overdosage may manifest with accentuation of adverse effects, but virtually no information is available thus far. Manage with general supportive and symptomatic measures, and consider hemodialysis in extreme cases

Indications

Short-term treatment of endoscopically proven active duodenal or benign gastric ulcer

Long-term therapy to reduce the incidence of recurrent duodenal or gastric ulcer

Short-term relief of symptomatic gastroesophageal reflux

Treatment of hypersecretory disorders of the gastrointestinal tract such as Zollinger-Ellison syndrome and systemic mastocytosis

Management of erosive esophagitis

Unlabeled Uses. Control of upper gastrointestinal bleeding and treatment of recurrent postoperative ulcer

Pharmacokinetics

Onset of IV Action. Less than 15 minutes

Peak IV Effects. Within 15 minutes

Duration of Action. 6–8 hours after single 50-mg IV dose

Elimination Half-Life. 1.7–3.2 hours

Metabolism. Via liver with renal elimination

Ranitidine Hydrochloride (Zantac)

Dosing Information

Intermittent IV Infusion. 50 mg diluted in 20–100 mL of 5% dextrose or 0.9% sodium chloride solution over 5–20 minutes. May repeat every 6–8 hours as necessary

Continuous IV Infusion. 150 mg diluted in 250 mL of 5% dextrose or 0.9% sodium chloride solution. Infuse at 6.25 mg/hr over 24 hours

Hypersecretory Disorders. 1 mg/kg/hr over 24 hours

Maximum Infusion Rate. 2.5 mg/kg/hr or 220 mg/hr

Maximum Infusion Dose. 400 mg/24 hrs

Titration Guidelines

Suggested Regimen. Adjust infusion by 6.25 mg/hr as necessary

Hypersecretory Disorders. Adjust infusion by 0.5 mg/kg/hr as required

Potential Drug Interactions

Potentiation of Ranitidine Effects. Propantheline bromide

Antagonism of Ranitidine Effects. Aluminum and magnesium hydroxide

Principal Adverse Effects

CNS. Headache, dizziness, insomnia, malaise, somnolence, and vertigo

CV. Bradycardia, heart block, asystole, ventricular ectopy, and tachycardia

GI. Nausea, vomiting, constipation, pancreatitis, abdominal pain, and abnormal liver function tests

Heme. Pancytopenia and aplastic anemia

Musculoskeletal. Myalgias, arthralgias

Dermatological. Rash, urticaria, erythema multiforme, and alopecia

Miscellaneous. Elevation of serum creatinine, anaphylaxis, blurred vision, hypersensitivity reactions

How Supplied

0.5 mg/mL—premixed solution of 50 mg in 100 mL 0.45% sodium chloride

25 mg/mL—2-mL vials and syringes of 50 mg
10-mL vials of 250 mg
40-mL vials of 1000 mg

Ranitidine Hydrochloride (Zantac) 150 mg in 250 mL

■ **Infusion Rate in mL/hr (pump setting)** ■ **Drug Dose in mg/hr**

mL/hr	mg/hr	mL/hr	mg/hr	mL/hr	mg/hr	mL/hr	mg/hr	mL/hr	mg/hr	mL/hr	mg/hr
1	0.6	21	12.6	41	24.6	61	36.6	81	48.6	101	60.6
2	1.2	22	13.2	42	25.2	62	37.2	82	49.2	102	61.2
3	1.8	23	13.8	43	25.8	63	37.8	83	49.8	103	61.8
4	2.4	24	14.4	44	26.4	64	38.4	84	50.4	104	62.4
5	3.0	25	15.0	45	27.0	65	39.0	85	51.0	105	63.0
6	3.6	26	15.6	46	27.6	66	39.6	86	51.6	106	63.6
7	4.2	27	16.2	47	28.2	67	40.2	87	52.2	107	64.2
8	4.8	28	16.8	48	28.8	68	40.8	88	52.8	108	64.8
9	5.4	29	17.4	49	29.4	69	41.4	89	53.4	109	65.4
10	6.0	30	18.0	50	30.0	70	42.0	90	54.0	110	66.0
11	6.6	31	18.6	51	30.6	71	42.6	91	54.6	111	66.6
12	7.2	32	19.2	52	31.2	72	43.2	92	55.2	112	67.2
13	7.8	33	19.8	53	31.8	73	43.8	93	55.8	113	67.8
14	8.4	34	20.4	54	32.4	74	44.4	94	56.4	114	68.4
15	9.0	35	21.0	55	33.0	75	45.0	95	57.0	115	69.0
16	9.6	36	21.6	56	33.6	76	45.6	96	57.6	116	69.6
17	10.2	37	22.2	57	34.2	77	46.2	97	58.2	117	70.2
18	10.8	38	22.8	58	34.8	78	46.8	98	58.8	118	70.8
19	11.4	39	23.4	59	35.4	79	47.4	99	59.4	119	71.4
20	12.0	40	24.0	60	36.0	80	48.0	100	60.0	120	72.0

DRUG DOSE in mg/kg/hr

Patient's Weight kg / lbs	40 / 88	45 / 99	50 / 110	55 / 121	60 / 132	65 / 143	70 / 154	75 / 165	80 / 176	85 / 187	90 / 198	95 / 209	100 / 220	105 / 231	110 / 242
Infusion Rate in mL/hr															
5	0.08	0.07	0.06	0.05	0.05	0.05	0.04	0.04	0.04	0.04	0.03	0.03	0.03	0.03	0.03
10	0.15	0.13	0.12	0.11	0.10	0.09	0.09	0.08	0.08	0.07	0.07	0.06	0.06	0.06	0.05
15	0.22	0.20	0.18	0.16	0.15	0.14	0.13	0.12	0.11	0.11	0.10	0.09	0.09	0.09	0.08
20	0.30	0.27	0.24	0.22	0.20	0.18	0.17	0.16	0.15	0.14	0.13	0.13	0.12	0.11	0.11
25	0.38	0.33	0.30	0.27	0.25	0.23	0.21	0.20	0.19	0.18	0.17	0.16	0.15	0.14	0.14
30	0.45	0.40	0.36	0.33	0.30	0.28	0.26	0.24	0.22	0.21	0.20	0.19	0.18	0.17	0.16
35	0.52	0.47	0.42	0.38	0.35	0.32	0.30	0.28	0.26	0.25	0.23	0.22	0.21	0.20	0.19
40	0.60	0.53	0.48	0.44	0.40	0.37	0.34	0.32	0.30	0.28	0.27	0.25	0.24	0.23	0.22
45	0.68	0.60	0.54	0.49	0.45	0.42	0.39	0.36	0.34	0.32	0.30	0.28	0.27	0.26	0.25
50	0.75	0.67	0.60	0.55	0.50	0.46	0.43	0.40	0.38	0.35	0.33	0.32	0.30	0.29	0.27
55	0.82	0.73	0.66	0.60	0.55	0.51	0.47	0.44	0.41	0.39	0.37	0.35	0.33	0.31	0.30
60	0.90	0.80	0.72	0.65	0.60	0.55	0.51	0.48	0.45	0.42	0.40	0.38	0.36	0.34	0.33
65	0.98	0.87	0.78	0.71	0.65	0.60	0.56	0.52	0.49	0.46	0.43	0.41	0.39	0.37	0.35
70	1.05	0.93	0.84	0.76	0.70	0.65	0.60	0.56	0.52	0.49	0.47	0.44	0.42	0.40	0.38
75	1.13	1.00	0.90	0.82	0.75	0.69	0.64	0.60	0.56	0.53	0.50	0.47	0.45	0.43	0.41
80	1.20	1.07	0.96	0.87	0.80	0.74	0.69	0.64	0.60	0.56	0.53	0.51	0.48	0.46	0.44
85	1.28	1.13	1.02	0.93	0.85	0.78	0.73	0.68	0.64	0.60	0.57	0.54	0.51	0.49	0.46
90	1.35	1.20	1.08	0.98	0.90	0.83	0.77	0.72	0.68	0.64	0.60	0.57	0.54	0.51	0.49
95	1.43	1.27	1.14	1.04	0.95	0.88	0.81	0.76	0.71	0.67	0.63	0.60	0.57	0.54	0.52
100	1.50	1.33	1.20	1.09	1.00	0.92	0.86	0.80	0.75	0.71	0.67	0.63	0.60	0.57	0.55
105	1.58	1.40	1.26	1.15	1.05	0.97	0.90	0.84	0.79	0.74	0.70	0.66	0.63	0.60	0.57
110	1.65	1.47	1.32	1.20	1.10	1.02	0.94	0.88	0.82	0.78	0.73	0.69	0.66	0.63	0.60
115	1.73	1.53	1.38	1.25	1.15	1.06	0.99	0.92	0.86	0.81	0.77	0.73	0.69	0.66	0.63
120	1.80	1.60	1.44	1.31	1.20	1.11	1.03	0.96	0.90	0.85	0.80	0.76	0.72	0.69	0.65

Sodium Bicarbonate

Pharmacology

Hypertonic alkalinizing agent that dissociates to provide bicarbonate ion. Each gram can neutralize 12 mEq of acid

Conjugate base component with carbonic acid (20 : 1 ratio), which constitutes the major extracellular buffer in humans

Increases plasma bicarbonate, buffers excess hydrogen ions, raises urine pH, and may elevate blood pH to correct consequences of metabolic acidosis

May produce hypokalemia via intracellular potassium shift, paradoxic spinal fluid acidosis, hyperosmolarity and hypernatremia, inactivation of exogenous catecholamines, tissue hypoxia because of shift in oxyhemoglobin dissociation curve, extracellular alkalosis, or central venous acidosis

1 g of sodium bicarbonate provides 11.9 mEq of sodium and 11.9 mEq of bicarbonate

Administrative Guidelines

Administer infusion via precision control device

Carefully monitor ECG, vital signs, electrolytes, and acid-base status

Correct hypokalemia, hypochloremia, and hypocalcemia, if possible, before use

Employ central line, if possible, or large vein

Do not attempt complete correction of bicarbonate deficit during the first 24 hours of therapy

Do not admix with calcium, norepinephrine, or dobutamine

Dilute to isotonicity (1–5%), if possible, before use. When only 7.5% or 8.4% solution is available, dilute 1:1 in 5% dextrose in water (USP) before administration

Avoid tissue extravasation because cellulitis, ulceration, sloughing, and necrosis may occur. When extravasation is noted, elevate site, apply warmth, and

(continued below)

Indications

Alkalinization of the serum in conditions associated with significant metabolic acidosis, including severe renal failure, hypoperfusion syndromes caused by shock or dehydration, primary lactic acidosis, and during extracorporeal bypass

Management of drug intoxications complicated by acidosis, such as salicylates, methyl alcohol, phenobarbital, and lithium

Augmentation of urinary pH to aid in solubility and excretion of weak acids and blood pigments arising from hemolytic syndromes

Adjunctive therapy to correct hyperkalemia in renal failure or severe bicarbonate wasting syndromes caused by diarrhea or gastrointestinal disorders

Additive to raise pH in solutions prone to causing phlebitis

Discretionary use during advanced cardiac life support, especially with preexisting hyperkalemia, prolonged

(continued on page 258)

discontinue infusion. Consider local injection of lidocaine or hyaluronidase

Avoid rapid infusion because hypernatremia, alkalosis, irritability, and tetany may ensue

Contraindicated in patients with respiratory and metabolic alkalosis; patients with hypocalcemia in whom alkalosis may precipitate tetany; patients with hypertension, seizures, or congestive heart failure; those on diuretics known to cause hypochloremic alkalosis; and patients with excessive chloride loss from vomiting or gastrointestinal suctioning

Use with caution in patients in edematous or salt-retaining states, patients with renal insufficiency, those receiving corticosteroids or corticotropin, elderly or debilitated patients, patients in postoperative states, and those with conditions predisposing to heart failure

Overdosage typically produces alkalosis and may produce hyperirritability, tetany, and seizures. Consider rebreathing mask or bag, parenteral calcium gluconate for tetany, and potassium chloride for hypokalemia. Severe alkalosis may require 2.14% ammonium chloride infusion except in those with hepatic disease cardiac arrest, or *documented* severe metabolic acidosis (usually pH less than 7.2 or bicarbonate less than 8 mEq/L) unresponsive to standard resuscitative measures

The role of bicarbonate therapy in diabetic acidosis is controversial

Pharmacokinetics

Onset of Action. Immediately

Metabolism. Virtually all of the bicarbonate ion filtered by the glomerulus is reabsorbed

Dosing Information

Cardiac Arrest (When Indicated). 1 mEq/kg IV load initially, then 0.5 mEq/kg IV push at 10-minute intervals guided by clinical response, blood gas analysis, bicarbonate measurements, and the following equation:

mEq sodium bicarbonate =
0.3 x body weight (kg) x base deficit (mEq/L)

Severe Metabolic Acidosis. 90–180 mEq/L at a rate up to 1–1.5 L over the first hour

Non–Life-Threatening Acidosis. 2–5 mEq/kg infusion over 4–8 hours. Alternative estimated bicarbonate dose regimens include:

0.5 (L/kg) x body weight (kg) x desired increase in serum HCO_3 (mEq/L) = bicarbonate dose (mEq)

or

(continued on page 260)

Potential Drug Interactions

Possibly Potentiated by Sodium Bicarbonate. Flecainide, quinidine, sympathomimetics, anorexiants, mecamylamine

Possibly Antagonized by Sodium Bicarbonate. Lithium, chlorpropamide, methotrexate, tetracyclines, salicylates

Principal Adverse Effects

CNS. Altered consciousness, obtundation, seizures, coma, paradoxical spinal fluid acidosis, irritability, tetany

CV. Hypervolemia, congestive heart failure, edema, lactic acidosis

Dermatological. Skin sloughing, necrosis, and cellulitis at injection site

Miscellaneous. Hypernatremia, hyperosmolar states, hypokalemia, hypocalcemia, fever

Sodium Bicarbonate

0.5 (L/kg) x body weight (kg) x base deficit (mEq/L) = bicarbonate dose (mEq)

or

5 mEq/kg when plasma CO_2 content is unknown

Neutralizing Additive Solution. 1 vial of additive solution for each liter of parenteral solution

Titration Guideline

Suggested Regimen. Adjust infusion dose and duration based on clinical response and acid-base determinations. Approximately 50% base deficit reduction, pH of 7.2, or plasma CO_2 content greater than 20 mEq/L is usually sufficient

How Supplied

Neutralizing Additive Solution

4% (0.48 mEq/mL)—5-mL vials of 2.4 mEq

4.2% (0.50 mEq/mL)—5-mL vials of 2.5 mEq

(continued below)

Parenteral Injection

4.2% (0.5 mEq/mL)—5-mL syringes of 2.5 mEq
10-mL syringes of 5 mEq

7.5% (0.9 mEq/mL)—50-mL ampuls, syringes, and vial of 44.6 mEq
200-mL bulk package of 179 mEq

8.4% (1 mEq/mL)—10-mL syringes of 10 mEq
50-mL vials and syringes of 50 mEq

Parenteral Infusion

5% (0.6 mEq/mL)—500-mL solution of 297.5 mEq

Sodium Bicarbonate

298 mEq in 500 mL

■ Infusion Rate in mL/hr (pump setting) ■ Drug Dose in mEq/hr

mL/hr	mEq/hr	mL/hr	mEq/hr	mL/hr	mEq/hr	mL/hr	mEq/hr	mL/hr	mEq/hr	mL/hr	mEq/hr
1	0.6	21	12.5	41	24.4	61	36.3	81	48.2	101	60.1
2	1.2	22	13.1	42	25.0	62	36.9	82	48.8	102	60.7
3	1.8	23	13.7	43	25.6	63	37.5	83	49.4	103	61.3
4	2.4	24	14.3	44	26.2	64	38.1	84	50.0	104	61.9
5	3.0	25	14.9	45	26.8	65	38.7	85	50.6	105	62.5
6	3.6	26	15.5	46	27.4	66	39.3	86	51.2	106	63.1
7	4.2	27	16.1	47	28.0	67	39.9	87	51.8	107	63.7
8	4.8	28	16.7	48	28.6	68	40.5	88	52.4	108	64.3
9	5.4	29	17.3	49	29.2	69	41.1	89	53.0	109	64.9
10	6.0	30	17.9	50	29.8	70	41.7	90	53.6	110	65.5
11	6.5	31	18.4	51	30.3	71	42.2	91	54.1	111	66.0
12	7.1	32	19.0	52	30.9	72	42.8	92	54.7	112	66.6
13	7.7	33	19.6	53	31.5	73	43.4	93	55.3	113	67.2
14	8.3	34	20.2	54	32.1	74	44.0	94	55.9	114	67.8
15	8.9	35	20.8	55	32.7	75	44.6	95	56.5	115	68.4
16	9.5	36	21.4	56	33.3	76	45.2	96	57.1	116	69.0
17	10.1	37	22.0	57	33.9	77	45.8	97	57.7	117	69.6
18	10.7	38	22.6	58	34.5	78	46.4	98	58.3	118	70.2
19	11.3	39	23.2	59	35.1	79	47.0	99	58.9	119	70.8
20	11.9	40	23.8	60	35.7	80	47.6	100	59.5	120	71.4

Infusion Rate in mL/hr (pump setting)	Drug Dose in mEq/hr	Infusion Rate in mL/hr (pump setting)	Drug Dose in mEq/hr	Infusion Rate in mL/hr (pump setting)	Drug Dose in mEq/hr	Infusion Rate in mL/hr (pump setting)	Drug Dose in mEq/hr	Infusion Rate in mL/hr (pump setting)	Drug Dose in mEq/hr	Infusion Rate in mL/hr (pump setting)	Drug Dose in mEq/hr
1	1.00	21	21.00	41	41.00	61	61.00	81	81.00	101	101.00
2	2.00	22	22.00	42	42.00	62	62.00	82	82.00	102	102.00
3	3.00	23	23.00	43	43.00	63	63.00	83	83.00	103	103.00
4	4.00	24	24.00	44	44.00	64	64.00	84	84.00	104	104.00
5	5.00	25	25.00	45	45.00	65	65.00	85	85.00	105	105.00
6	6.00	26	26.00	46	46.00	66	66.00	86	86.00	106	106.00
7	7.00	27	27.00	47	47.00	67	67.00	87	87.00	107	107.00
8	8.00	28	28.00	48	48.00	68	68.00	88	88.00	108	108.00
9	9.00	29	29.00	49	49.00	69	69.00	89	89.00	109	109.00
10	10.00	30	30.00	50	50.00	70	70.00	90	90.00	110	110.00
11	11.00	31	31.00	51	51.00	71	71.00	91	91.00	111	111.00
12	12.00	32	32.00	52	52.00	72	72.00	92	92.00	112	112.00
13	13.00	33	33.00	53	53.00	73	73.00	93	93.00	113	113.00
14	14.00	34	34.00	54	54.00	74	74.00	94	94.00	114	114.00
15	15.00	35	35.00	55	55.00	75	75.00	95	95.00	115	115.00
16	16.00	36	36.00	56	56.00	76	76.00	96	96.00	116	116.00
17	17.00	37	37.00	57	57.00	77	77.00	97	97.00	117	117.00
18	18.00	38	38.00	58	58.00	78	78.00	98	98.00	118	118.00
19	19.00	39	39.00	59	59.00	79	79.00	99	99.00	119	119.00
20	20.00	40	40.00	60	60.00	80	80.00	100	100.00	120	120.00

Sodium Nitroprusside (Nipride)

Pharmacology

Potent, rapid-acting peripheral vasodilator with direct relaxation effects on vascular smooth muscle—other smooth muscle tissues not affected

Dilates venous (capacitance) vessels to a greater extent than arterial (resistance) vessels; also dilates coronary arteries and may produce renal vasodilation in hypertensive subjects

Reduces venous return (preload) and lowers pulmonary capillary wedge and left ventricular end diastolic pressures; also reduces systemic vascular resistance (afterload) and lowers systolic and mean arterial pressures

Variable effects on cardiac performance but usually decreases myocardial oxygen consumption

Tachyphylaxis may occur

Administrative Guidelines

Administer infusion via precision control device

Continuously monitor ECG and blood pressure; carefully follow respirations, acid-base status, and venous oxygen

Monitor hemodynamics, when indicated, with Swan-Ganz catheter

Protect solutions from light, heat, and moisture—wrap infusion solution with opaque material but ***not*** drip chamber or tubing

Reconstitute only with 5% dextrose injection USP and dilute in at least 250 mL before infusion—reconstituted solution is stable up to 24 hours

Faint brownish tint to solution is normal—discard if strongly colored or particulate matter observed

Do not admix with any other drugs

Correct any underlying hypovolemia and anemia, if possible, before use

(continued below)

Indications

Immediate reduction of blood pressure in patients with hypertensive crises

Controlled hypotension during surgery to minimize bleeding

Unlabeled Uses. Management of congestive heart failure to improve hemodynamics; adjunct to beta-blockers in patients with aortic dissection

Pharmacokinetics

Onset of Action. 30–60 seconds

Peak Effects. Usually 1–2 minutes

Duration of Action. 1–10 minutes

Plasma Half-Life. Approximately 2 minutes

Metabolism. Via intraerythrocytic reaction with hemoglobin to form cyanmethemoglobin and cyanide

Determine daily thiocyanate levels after 24 hours infusion if anuric patients are receiving at least 1 μg/kg/min or those with normal renal function are receiving at least 3 μg/kg/min

Contraindicated in those with known hypersensitivity, or compensatory hypertension; in patients with aortic coarctation or arteriovenous shunting, congenital (Lieber's) optic atrophy, tobacco amblyopia, or known cerebrovascular insufficiency; or during surgery of moribund patients

Use with caution in elderly patients; those with renal or hepatic failure, hypothyroidism, hypovolemia, hyponatremia, vitamin B_{12} deficiency, uncorrected anemia, or preexisting increased intracranial pressure; and those receiving antihypertensive medications

Overdosage may manifest as hypotension, methemoglobinemia, or cyanide or thiocyanate toxicity. These may occur rapidly without premonitory signs and symptoms. Incidence increases with higher doses (>3 μg/kg/min) and more prolonged use (>24 hours)

Hypotension—discontinue infusion, place patient in Trendelenburg position, and consider other causes

(continued on page 266)

for reduced pressure if improvement is not observed within 10 minutes. Epinephrine may be indicated in extreme situations

Thiocyanate toxicity—may manifest with tinnitus, meiosis, or hyperreflexia with serum levels of 60 μg/mL. May be lethal at serum levels of 200 μg/mL. Discontinue infusion and consider hemodialysis

Methemoglobinemia—typically manifests as impaired oxygen delivery despite adequate arterial oxygen tension and cardiac output. Blood is chocolate-brown in appearance. Rarely seen unless patients are receiving 10 μg/kg/min for 16 hours or 10 mg/kg cumulative daily dose. Administer 1–2 mg/kg methylene blue IV over several minutes

Cyanide toxicity—frequently manifests with metabolic acidosis, CNS disturbances, drug tolerance, venous hyperoxemia, faint pulse, dilated pupils, areflexia, and shallow breathing. Death may ensue within 1 hour. Immediately discontinue

(continued below)

infusion, measure cyanide levels and blood gases, but do ***not*** wait for cyanide levels to initiate treatment. Begin amyl nitrite inhalation every 15–30 seconds until 3% sodium nitrite solution can be prepared. Administer 4–6 mg/kg 3% sodium nitrite slow IV injection over 2–4 minutes. Thereafter, if needed, begin 25% solution of sodium thiosulfate at a dose of 150–200 mg/kg IV (approximately 50 mL of the 25% solution)—may repeat sodium nitrite and thiosulfate regimen at one-half the initial recommended doses every 2 hours. There is no established role for hemodialysis

Sodium Nitroprusside (Nipride)

Dosing Information

Initial Infusion Rate. 0.3 μg/kg/min

Maintenance Infusion Range. 0.3–3 μg/kg/min

Maximum Infusion Rate. 10 μg/kg/min

Discontinue infusion if blood pressure has not been adequately controlled after 10 minutes of infusion at maximal dose of 10 μg/kg/min. Lethal cyanide toxicity can develop in less than 1 hour at this dose

Infusion rates greater than 2 μg/kg/min produce cyanide faster than the body can dispose of it

Generally, infuse at rates less than 3 μg/kg/min with normal renal function and at 1 μg/kg/min in anuric patients

Titration Guideline

Suggested Regimen. Adjust infusion by 0.15 μg/kg/min every 5–10 minutes as required

Potential Drug Interactions

Potentiation of Nitroprusside Effects. Ganglionic blocking drugs, circulatory depressants, negative inotropic agents, antihypertensive drugs, inhalational anesthetics

Principal Adverse Effects

CNS. Dizziness, diaphoresis, headache, restlessness, apprehension, muscle twitching, increased intracranial pressure, respiratory depression, and coma

CV. Palpitations, hypotension, bradycardia, tachycardia, chest pain, ECG changes

GI. Nausea, vomiting, abdominal pain, ileus

Dermatological. Irritation and venous streaking at injection site, rash

Heme. Decreased platelet aggregation and methemoglobinemia

Miscellaneous. Cyanide and thiocyanate toxicity, flushing, hypothyroidism

Toxic Serum Levels

Thiocyanate. 60 μg/mL or greater

Methemoglobin. 10% or greater

How Supplied

10 mg/mL—2-mL vials of 20 mg
5-mL vials of 50 mg

Sodium Nitroprusside (Nipride) 100 mg in 500 mL

■ **Infusion Rate in mL/hr (pump setting)** ■ **Drug Dose in μg/min**

mL/hr	μg/min	mL/hr	μg/min	mL/hr	μg/min	mL/hr	μg/min	mL/hr	μg/min	mL/hr	μg/min
1	3	21	70	41	137	61	203	81	270	101	337
2	7	22	73	42	140	62	207	82	273	102	340
3	10	23	77	43	143	63	210	83	277	103	343
4	13	24	80	44	147	64	213	84	280	104	347
5	17	25	83	45	150	65	217	85	283	105	350
6	20	26	87	46	153	66	220	86	287	106	353
7	23	27	90	47	157	67	223	87	290	107	357
8	27	28	93	48	160	68	227	88	293	108	360
9	30	29	97	49	163	69	230	89	297	109	363
10	33	30	100	50	167	70	233	90	300	110	367
11	37	31	103	51	170	71	237	91	303	111	370
12	40	32	107	52	173	72	240	92	307	112	373
13	43	33	110	53	177	73	243	93	310	113	377
14	47	34	113	54	180	74	247	94	313	114	380
15	50	35	117	55	183	75	250	95	317	115	383
16	53	36	120	56	187	76	253	96	320	116	387
17	57	37	123	57	190	77	257	97	323	117	390
18	60	38	127	58	193	78	260	98	327	118	393
19	63	39	130	59	197	79	263	99	330	119	397
20	67	40	133	60	200	80	267	100	333	120	400

DRUG DOSE in μg/kg/min

Infusion Rate in mL/hr	Patient's Weight kg / lbs: 40 / 88	45 / 99	50 / 110	55 / 121	60 / 132	65 / 143	70 / 154	75 / 165	80 / 176	85 / 187	90 / 198	95 / 209	100 / 220	105 / 231	110 / 242
5	0.4	0.4	0.3	0.3	0.3	0.3	0.2	0.2	0.2	0.2	0.2	0.2	0.2	0.2	0.2
10	0.8	0.7	0.7	0.6	0.6	0.5	0.5	0.4	0.4	0.4	0.4	0.4	0.3	0.3	0.3
15	1.2	1.1	1.0	0.9	0.8	0.8	0.7	0.7	0.6	0.6	0.6	0.5	0.5	0.5	0.5
20	1.7	1.5	1.3	1.2	1.1	1.0	1.0	0.9	0.8	0.8	0.7	0.7	0.7	0.6	0.6
25	2.1	1.9	1.7	1.5	1.4	1.3	1.2	1.1	1.0	1.0	0.9	0.9	0.8	0.8	0.8
30	2.5	2.2	2.0	1.8	1.7	1.5	1.4	1.3	1.2	1.2	1.1	1.1	1.0	1.0	0.9
35	2.9	2.6	2.3	2.1	1.9	1.8	1.7	1.6	1.5	1.4	1.3	1.2	1.2	1.1	1.1
40	3.3	3.0	2.7	2.4	2.2	2.1	1.9	1.8	1.7	1.6	1.5	1.4	1.3	1.3	1.2
45	3.7	3.3	3.0	2.7	2.5	2.3	2.1	2.0	1.9	1.8	1.7	1.6	1.5	1.4	1.4
50	4.2	3.7	3.3	3.0	2.8	2.6	2.4	2.2	2.1	2.0	1.9	1.8	1.7	1.6	1.5
55	4.6	4.1	3.7	3.3	3.1	2.8	2.6	2.4	2.3	2.2	2.0	1.9	1.8	1.7	1.7
60	5.0	4.4	4.0	3.6	3.3	3.1	2.9	2.7	2.5	2.4	2.2	2.1	2.0	1.9	1.8
65	5.4	4.8	4.3	3.9	3.6	3.3	3.1	2.9	2.7	2.5	2.4	2.3	2.2	2.1	2.0
70	5.8	5.2	4.7	4.2	3.9	3.6	3.3	3.1	2.9	2.7	2.6	2.5	2.3	2.2	2.1
75	6.2	5.6	5.0	4.5	4.2	3.8	3.6	3.3	3.1	2.9	2.8	2.6	2.5	2.4	2.3
80	6.7	5.9	5.3	4.8	4.4	4.1	3.8	3.6	3.3	3.1	3.0	2.8	2.7	2.5	2.4
85	7.1	6.3	5.7	5.2	4.7	4.4	4.0	3.8	3.5	3.3	3.1	3.0	2.8	2.7	2.6
90	7.5	6.7	6.0	5.5	5.0	4.6	4.3	4.0	3.7	3.5	3.3	3.2	3.0	2.9	2.7
95	7.9	7.0	6.3	5.8	5.3	4.9	4.5	4.2	4.0	3.7	3.5	3.3	3.2	3.0	2.9
100	8.3	7.4	6.7	6.1	5.6	5.1	4.8	4.4	4.2	3.9	3.7	3.5	3.3	3.2	3.0
105	8.7	7.8	7.0	6.4	5.8	5.4	5.0	4.7	4.4	4.1	3.9	3.7	3.5	3.3	3.2
110	9.2	8.1	7.3	6.7	6.1	5.6	5.2	4.9	4.6	4.3	4.1	3.9	3.7	3.5	3.3
115	9.6	8.5	7.7	7.0	6.4	5.9	5.5	5.1	4.8	4.5	4.3	4.0	3.8	3.7	3.5
120	10.0	8.9	8.0	7.3	6.7	6.2	5.7	5.3	5.0	4.7	4.4	4.2	4.0	3.8	3.6

Streptokinase (Kabikinase, Streptase)

Pharmacology

Thrombolytic protein derived from group C beta-hemolytic streptococci—highly antigenic

Mechanism of action involves formation of activator complex with plasminogen, which converts residual plasminogen to plasmin. Subsequently, plasmin degrades fibrin, fibrinogen, and other procoagulant proteins

Site of action includes endogenous lysis by diffusion of activator complex into the thrombus and exogenous lysis of thrombus by circulating plasmin

Effects of streptokinase may be antagonized by circulating plasmin inhibitors, including alpha$_2$-antiplasmin and macroglobulin

May produce additional anticoagulant effects by causing hyperplasminemia and depletion of factors I, V, and VIII

(continued below)

Administrative Guidelines

Administer infusion via precision control device

Continuously monitor ECG and carefully follow vital signs during infusion

When preparing infusions, do not add other medications to the vial and reconstitute with 0.9% sodium chloride or 5% dextrose injection. Gently tilt and roll vial, but avoid shaking. Discard solution if flocculation observed

Determine thrombin time, hematocrit, platelet count, cardiac enzymes, prothrombin time, activated partial thromboplastin time (APTT), and fibrinogen levels, if possible, **before** initiating therapy. Do not begin streptokinase therapy in cases of a suspected bleeding diathesis unless the thrombin time and APTT are less than twice control values

Measure thrombin time, APTT, fibrinogen, and prothrombin time 4 hours after beginning prolonged infusion therapy. Failure of these parameters to be

(continued below)

Decreases plasma fibrinogen, blood viscosity, and red blood cell aggregation, thereby promoting collateral blood flow

Altered platelet function and indirect reduction of peripheral vascular resistance have also been noted

Activity is standardized and expressed in International Units (IU) based on in vitro fibrin clot lysis within 10 minutes

altered beyond 1.5 times control values indicates excessive resistance, and the infusion should be terminated. With prolonged infusions, consider thrombin times every 12 hours as well as before crossover therapy with heparin

Avoid intramuscular injections before, during, and 24 hours after streptokinase therapy. Do not attempt central venous access or arterial puncture during this period unless absolutely essential (upper extremity sites are preferred)

Minimize performance of venipuncture and handling of patient

Compress venipuncture sites for up to 30 minutes to control minor bleeding, apply a pressure dressing, and check site frequently

Apply local pressure to minor surface bleeding areas as necessary but do not alter the infusion dose with superficial bleeding. Immediately discontinue therapy, however, if serious external or internal hemorrhage is observed

(continued on page 274)

Streptokinase (Kabikinase, Streptase)

Indications

Acute (within 7 days), massive, diagnostically confirmed pulmonary emboli associated with significant lobar obstruction or unstable hemodynamics

Intravenous or intracoronary lysis of acute evolving transmural myocardial infarction—initiate therapy preferably within 6 hours of symptom onset

Acute (preferably within 7 days) arterial emboli or thrombi **not** originating from a left heart focus

Extensive, **diagnostically confirmed,** acute deep vein thrombosis—initiate therapy preferably within 3 days of confirmation, although intervention begun within 2 weeks may occasionally be useful

Clearance of occluded arteriovenous cannulae only when obstructed by clotted blood or fibrin

Unlabeled Uses. Retinal vessel thrombosis and chronic arterial occlusions

It is unnecessary to determine streptococcal resistance levels routinely before treatment. Consider 100-unit intradermal test dose in acutely ill patients who would be adversely affected by allergic responses and interpret after 15–20 minutes. Test doses may also be helpful when there is a history of streptokinase allergy, recent streptococcal infection, or treatment with streptokinase within 6 months

Efficacy and bleeding risk do not directly correlate with laboratory parameters of the lytic state

Contraindicated in patients with known hypersensitivity, active internal bleeding, severe uncontrolled hypertension, intracranial tumor, aneurysm or arteriovenous malformation, intracranial or intraspinal surgery or trauma, and cerebrovascular accident within the previous 2 months

Use with extreme caution in patients with hypertension exceeding 180 mmHg systolic or 110 mmHg diastolic pressure and recent (within 10 days) serious trauma, major surgery, organ biopsy,

(continued below)

Pharmacokinetics

Plasma Half-Life. 18–83 minutes depending on amount of neutralizing streptococcal antibodies

Metabolism. Via the reticuloendothelial system and streptococcal antibodies

gastrointestinal bleeding, obstetrical delivery, or puncture of a noncompressible artery

Use with caution in patients following cardiopulmonary resuscitation or minor trauma (within 10 days); in patients with suspected mural thrombus, pregnancy, hemorrhagic diabetic retinopathy, cerebrovascular disease, acute pericarditis, subacute bacterial endocarditis, septic thrombophlebitis or occluded arteriovenous cannula at the site of serious infection, severe hepatic or renal disease, or atrial fibrillation; in conditions associated with increased bleeding risk; and in those over 75 years of age

Overdosage may manifest with severe hemorrhage. Provide general supportive measures and fluid resuscitate with volume expanders other than dextran. Transfuse with packed red blood cells, fresh frozen plasma, and cryoprecipitate as needed. Although unproven, IV aminocaproic acid may be efficacious in life-threatening cases

Streptokinase (Kabikinase, Streptase)

Dosing Information

Pulmonary Emboli. 250,000 units IV loading dose over 30 minutes, then 100,000 units/hr for 24 hours

Arterial Embolism or Thrombosis. 250,000 units IV loading dose over 30 minutes, then 100,000 units/hr for 24–72 hours

Deep Vein Thrombosis. 250,000 units IV loading dose over 30 minutes, then 100,000 units/hr for 72 hours. To prevent recurrent thrombosis, heparin infusion without a loading dose is recommended after the thrombin time has decreased to less than twice the control value

(continued below)

Potential Drug Interactions

Potentiation of Streptokinase Effects. Heparin, oral anticoagulants, aspirin, dipyridamole, indomethacin, phenylbutazone, sulfinpyrazone, ticlopidine

Antagonism of Streptokinase Effects. Aminocaproic acid

Acute Myocardial Infarction

Intracoronary. 20,000 units bolus, then 2000 units/min for up to 60 minutes until artery is maximally opened. Alternatively, 2000–5000 units/min infusion without a bolus has been employed

Intravenous. 1.5 million units over 60 minutes to prevent recurrent thrombosis. Pretreatment with 100 mg IV hydrocortisone or 50 mg IV diphenhydramine (Benadryl) may reduce allergic responses

Occluded Arteriovenous Cannulae. 250,000 units in 2-mL solution over 25–35 minutes via precision controlled device. Infuse into each line of cannulae, clamp for 2 hours, aspirate, and flush with saline before reconnecting

How Supplied

250,000 units—5-mL and 6.5-mL vials

600,000 units—5-mL vials

750,000 units—5-mL and 6.5-mL vials

1,500,000 units—6.5-mL vial and 50-mL infusion bottle

Principal Adverse Effects

CNS. Cerebrovascular hemorrhage and Guillain-Barré syndrome

Pulmonary. Pulmonary edema and emboli, bronchospasm

CV. Hypotension, bradycardia and reperfusion-related atrial and ventricular dysrhythmias, acute myocardial infarction

Heme. Spontaneous superficial and internal bleeding, unexplained decrease in hematocrit

Allergic. Urticaria, flushing, nausea, headache, angioneurotic edema, fever, pruritus, musculoskeletal pain, nephritis, vasculitis, serum sickness–like illness, anaphylaxis

Miscellaneous. Phlebitis, atheroemboli, elevated transaminase, altered sedimentation rate

Streptokinase (Kabikinase, Streptase) 750,000 units in 225 mL

■ **Infusion Rate in mL/hr (pump setting)** ■ **Drug Dose in units/hr**

mL/hr	units/hr	mL/hr	units/hr	mL/hr	units/hr	mL/hr	units/hr	mL/hr	units/hr	mL/hr	units/hr
1	3,333	21	70,000	41	136,667	61	203,333	81	270,000	101	336,667
2	6,667	22	73,333	42	140,000	62	206,667	82	273,333	102	340,000
3	10,000	23	76,667	43	143,333	63	210,000	83	276,667	103	343,333
4	13,333	24	80,000	44	146,667	64	213,333	84	280,000	104	346,667
5	16,667	25	83,333	45	150,000	65	216,667	85	283,333	105	350,000
6	20,000	26	86,667	46	153,333	66	220,000	86	286,667	106	353,333
7	23,333	27	90,000	47	156,667	67	223,333	87	290,000	107	356,667
8	26,667	28	93,333	48	160,000	68	226,667	88	293,333	108	360,000
9	30,000	29	96,667	49	163,333	69	230,000	89	296,667	109	363,333
10	33,333	30	100,000	50	166,667	70	233,333	90	300,000	110	366,667
11	36,667	31	103,333	51	170,000	71	236,667	91	303,333	111	370,000
12	40,000	32	106,667	52	173,333	72	240,000	92	306,667	112	373,333
13	43,333	33	110,000	53	176,667	73	243,333	93	310,000	113	376,667
14	46,667	34	113,333	54	180,000	74	246,667	94	313,333	114	380,000
15	50,000	35	116,667	55	183,333	75	250,000	95	316,667	115	383,333
16	53,333	36	120,000	56	186,667	76	253,333	96	320,000	116	386,667
17	56,667	37	123,333	57	190,000	77	256,667	97	323,333	117	390,000
18	60,000	38	126,667	58	193,333	78	260,000	98	326,667	118	393,333
19	63,333	39	130,000	59	196,667	79	263,333	99	330,000	119	396,667
20	66,667	40	133,333	60	200,000	80	266,667	100	333,333	120	400,000

Streptok[illegible]ase (Kabikinase, Streptase) 1,500,000 units in 22[illegible]

■ Infusion Rate in mL/hr (pump setting) ■ Drug Dose in units/hr

mL/hr	units/hr	mL/hr	units/hr	mL/hr	units/hr	mL/hr	units/hr	mL/hr	units/hr	mL/hr	units/hr
1	6,667	21	140,000	41	273,333	61	406,667	81	540,000	101	673,333
2	13,333	22	146,667	42	280,000	62	413,333	82	546,667	102	680,000
3	20,000	23	153,333	43	286,667	63	420,000	83	553,333	103	686,667
4	26,667	24	160,000	44	293,333	64	426,667	84	560,000	104	693,333
5	33,333	25	166,667	45	300,000	65	433,333	85	566,667	105	700,000
6	40,000	26	173,333	46	306,667	66	440,000	86	573,333	106	706,667
7	46,667	27	180,000	47	313,333	67	446,667	87	580,000	107	713,333
8	53,333	28	186,667	48	320,000	68	453,333	88	586,667	108	720,000
9	60,000	29	193,333	49	326,667	69	460,000	89	593,333	109	726,667
10	66,667	30	200,000	50	333,333	70	466,667	90	600,000	110	733,333
11	73,333	31	206,667	51	340,000	71	473,333	91	606,667	111	740,000
12	80,000	32	213,333	52	346,667	72	480,000	92	613,333	112	746,667
13	86,667	33	220,000	53	353,333	73	486,667	93	620,000	113	753,333
14	93,333	34	226,667	54	360,000	74	493,333	94	626,667	114	760,000
15	100,000	35	233,333	55	366,667	75	500,000	95	633,333	115	766,667
16	106,667	36	240,000	56	373,333	76	506,667	96	640,000	116	773,333
17	113,333	37	246,667	57	380,000	77	513,333	97	646,667	117	780,000
18	120,000	38	253,333	58	386,667	78	520,000	98	653,333	118	786,667
19	126,667	39	260,000	59	393,333	79	526,667	99	660,000	119	793,333
20	133,333	40	266,667	60	400,000	80	533,333	100	666,667	120	800,000

Theophylline Ethylenediamine (Aminophylline)

Pharmacology

Xanthine derivative, which is found in tea or synthetically manufactured—aminophylline is a theophylline compound combined with ethylenediamine

Competitively inhibits phosphodiesterase and thereby increases cyclic adenosine monophosphate—may also promote translocation of intracellular calcium, foster release of endogenous catecholamines, antagonize prostaglandins E_2 and $F_{2\alpha}$, and inhibit extracellular adenosine

Relaxes smooth muscle of respiratory tract, thus reducing bronchospasm; dilates pulmonary arterioles; lowers pulmonary pressure and carbon dioxide tension; and augments vital capacity, peak flow rates, and pulmonary blood flow

CNS stimulant with vasomotor and vagal effects at cortical, brain stem, and spinal cord levels. May alter blood pressure and heart rate, stimulate vomiting and seizures, eliminate neonatal apnea and Cheyne-Stokes respirations, and constrict cerebral vasculature

(continued below)

Administrative Guidelines

Administer infusion via precision control device

Carefully monitor the ECG and vital signs, and periodically determine serum drug levels

Do not admix with alkali-sensitive drugs and discard solution if crystals are observed

Decrease or discontinue infusion if serum levels are greater than 20 μg/mL—toxic manifestations are dose dependent

Initiate oral bronchodilator therapy as soon as feasible—generally within 4–6 hours after discontinuation of infusion

Smokers may require higher dosing because drug clearance is increased and plasma half-life decreased. Conversely, alcoholics and patients with renal hepatic or cardiac failure, respiratory infections, and chronic obstructive pulmonary disease may need reduced doses owing to prolongation of serum half-life

(continued below)

Produces dose-dependent positive inotropic and chronotropic cardiac response with variable effects on myocardial oxygen consumption. Directly vasodilates coronary vessels and enhances coronary blood flow. Also dilates systemic veins and arterioles with reduction in venous return and systemic vascular resistance. Blood pressure effects are variable depending on cardiac output response

Exhibits diuretic properties by renal vasodilation, increasing renal blood flow and glomerular filtration rate and inhibiting proximal tubular reabsorption of sodium and chloride

Stimulates skeletal muscle and gastric secretion and relaxes smooth muscle of the biliary and gastrointestinal tracts

May engender release of adrenal catecholamines; augment lipolysis, plasma free fatty acids, and basal metabolic rate; inhibit calcitonin; and potentiate corticotropin, parathyroid hormone–mediated calcium rise, and insulin secretion

Contraindicated in those with known hypersensitivity to xanthine, ethylenediamine, and sodium metabisulfite. May also be contraindicated with inappropriately treated underlying convulsive disorder or active peptic ulcer disease

Use with caution in those over 55 years of age, or in those with high fever, chronic obstructive pulmonary disease or cor pulmonale, influenza infection or recent vaccination, renal or hepatic dysfunction, peptic ulcer disease or acute gastritis, diabetes mellitus, glaucoma, hypertension, hyperthyroidism, heart failure, ischemic heart disease, hypoxemia, preexisting dysrhythmias, and alcoholism

Overdosage may manifest with tachydysrhythmias, anorexia, nausea, vomiting, agitation, headache, altered consciousness and behavior, tachypnea, fasciculations, diaphoresis, hyperthermia, convulsions, and cardiovascular collapse. Manage with supportive measures, including airway protection, correction of fluid and electrolytes, and periodic monitoring of serum theophylline levels until less than 20 μg/mL. Consider

(continued on page 282)

Theophylline Ethylenediamine (Aminophylline)

Indications

Bronchodilator in status asthmaticus refractory to epinephrine and symptomatic management of asthma and bronchospasm associated with emphysema or bronchitis

Unlabeled Uses. Adjunctive therapy for diuresis in patients on thiazides or carbonic anhydrase inhibitors; management of dyspnea and pulmonary congestion associated with heart failure; relief of Cheyne-Stokes–mediated apnea, apnea of infancy, and bronchospasm associated with cystic fibrosis; antagonism of adenosine or dipyridamole adverse effects during diagnostic stress testing

Pharmacokinetics

Onset of Action. Within 30 minutes

Peak Effects. Within 30–60 minutes

Duration of Action. Variable (hours)—not specified by manufacturer

Tissue (Elimination) Half-Life. 3–15 hours in nonsmokers; 4–5 hours in adult smokers

(continued below)

IV diazepam 0.1–0.3 mg/kg up to 10 mg for seizures and phenothiazines for hyperthermia. Gastric "dialysis" with 20–40 g of activated charcoal every 4 hours may accelerate removal. Charcoal hemoperfusion is indicated for serum levels greater than 60 μg/mL and may be advisable with levels greater than 30 μg/mL in patients with prolonged half-lives and severe symptoms. Hemodialysis may also be beneficial to enhance theophylline clearance

Metabolism. Principally via liver with renal excretion

Dosing Information

Acute Bronchospasm (IV Loading Dose). 4.7 mg/kg in 100–200 mL diluent over 20–30 minutes for patients ***not*** currently receiving theophylline

2.5 mg/kg in 100–200 mL diluent over 20–30 minutes for patients who ***are*** currently receiving theophylline. Ideally, defer loading dose until serum concentration is determined

Acute Bronchospasm (IV Maintenance Dose, First 12 Hours)

Young Adult Smokers. 0.79 mg/kg/hr

Nonsmoking Healthy Adults. 0.55 mg/kg/hr

Elderly Patients and Cor Pulmonale. 0.47 mg/kg/hr

Patients with Liver or Heart Failure. 0.39 mg/kg/hr

(continued on page 284)

Potential Drug Interactions

Potentiation of Theophylline Effects. Cimetidine, erythromycin, allopurinol, furosemide, influenza virus vaccine, thiabendazole, nonselective beta-blockers, calcium channel blockers, disulfiram, ephedrine, corticosteroids, oral contraceptives, interferon, isoniazid, macrolides, mexiletine, carbamazepine, quinolones, thyroid hormone, troleandomycin, ranitidine, tetracyclines, halothane, and high-carbohydrate/low-protein diet

Antagonism of Theophylline Effects. Cigarettes, marijuana, sympathomimetics, charcoal, barbiturates, aminoglutethimide, ketoconazole, rifampin, sulfinpyrazone, hydantoins, thioamines, loop diuretics, isoniazid, carbamezepine, and low-carbohydrate/high-protein diet

Possibly Potentiated by Theophylline. Ketamine, digitalis glycosides, sympathomimetics, and oral anticoagulants

Possibly Antagonized by Theophylline. Propofol, adenosine, benzodiazepines, lithium, nondepolarizing neuromuscular blockers, and dipyridamole

Theophylline Ethylenediamine (Aminophylline)

Acute Bronchospasm (IV Maintenance Dose After 12 Hours)

Young Adult Smokers. 0.63 mg/kg/hr

Nonsmoking Healthy Adults. 0.39 mg/kg/hr

Elderly Patients and Cor Pulmonale. 0.24 mg/kg/hr

Patients with Liver or Heart Failure. 0.08–0.16 mg/kg/hr

Maximum Infusion Rate. 0.7 mg/kg/hr

Maximum Daily Dose. 13 mg/kg/day or 900 mg

Do not exceed 20 mg/min IV administration, and reduce infusion rate if adverse effects are observed

Each 0.5 mg/kg (of lean body weight) IV loading dose raises serum theophylline levels approximately 1 μg/mL

Calculate dosage based on lean body mass because theophylline does ***not*** distribute into fatty tissue

Therapeutic Serum Levels

10–20 μg/mL

Principal Adverse Effects

CNS. Irritability, restlessness, dizziness, vertigo, agitation, nervousness, reflex hyperexcitability, headache, insomnia, stammering speech, muscle twitching, depression, and convulsions

Pulmonary. Respiratory arrest and tachypnea

CV. Palpitations, sinus tachycardia, ventricular dysrhythmias, chest pain, hypotension, circulatory collapse, bradycardia, and syncope

GI. Nausea, vomiting, anorexia, dyspepsia, reflux esophagitis, epigastric pain, hematemesis, reactivation of peptic ulcer disease, and diarrhea

Renal. Proteinuria, excessive diuresis, hematuria, and excretion of renal tubular cells

Allergic. Angioedema, rash, urticaria, flushing, exfoliative dermatitis, and pruritus

Miscellaneous. Hyperglycemia, hypercalcemia, hypokalemia, decreased bicarbonate, inappropriate antidiuretic hormone release; may increase serum AST (SGOT) values and falsely elevate serum uric acid

Titration Guideline

Suggested Regimen. Adjust infusion by 0.1 mg/kg/hr every 30–60 minutes as required

How Supplied

25 mg/mL—10-mL ampuls, vials, and syringes of 250 mg
20-mL ampuls, vials, and syringes of 500 mg
100-mL bulk vial of 2.5 g
200-mL bulk vial of 5.0 g

Theophylline Ethylenediamine (Aminophylline) 250 mg in 500 mL

DRUG DOSE in mg/kg/hr

Patient's Weight kg / lbs	40 / 88	45 / 99	50 / 110	55 / 121	60 / 132	65 / 143	70 / 154	75 / 165	80 / 176	85 / 187	90 / 198	95 / 209	100 / 220	105 / 231	110 / 242
Infusion Rate in mL/hr															
5	0.063	0.056	0.050	0.045	0.042	0.038	0.036	0.033	0.031	0.029	0.028	0.026	0.025	0.024	0.023
10	0.125	0.111	0.100	0.091	0.083	0.077	0.071	0.067	0.063	0.059	0.056	0.053	0.050	0.048	0.045
15	0.188	0.167	0.150	0.136	0.125	0.115	0.107	0.100	0.094	0.088	0.083	0.079	0.075	0.071	0.068
20	0.250	0.222	0.200	0.182	0.167	0.154	0.143	0.133	0.125	0.118	0.111	0.105	0.100	0.095	0.091
25	0.313	0.278	0.250	0.227	0.208	0.192	0.179	0.167	0.156	0.147	0.139	0.132	0.125	0.119	0.114
30	0.375	0.333	0.300	0.273	0.250	0.231	0.214	0.200	0.188	0.176	0.167	0.158	0.150	0.143	0.136
35	0.438	0.389	0.350	0.318	0.292	0.269	0.250	0.233	0.219	0.206	0.194	0.184	0.175	0.167	0.159
40	0.500	0.444	0.400	0.364	0.333	0.308	0.286	0.267	0.250	0.235	0.222	0.211	0.200	0.190	0.182
45	0.563	0.500	0.450	0.409	0.375	0.346	0.321	0.300	0.281	0.265	0.250	0.237	0.225	0.214	0.205
50	0.625	0.556	0.500	0.455	0.417	0.385	0.357	0.333	0.313	0.294	0.278	0.263	0.250	0.238	0.227
55	0.688	0.611	0.550	0.500	0.458	0.423	0.393	0.367	0.344	0.324	0.306	0.289	0.275	0.262	0.250
60	0.750	0.667	0.600	0.545	0.500	0.462	0.429	0.400	0.375	0.353	0.333	0.316	0.300	0.286	0.273
65	0.813	0.722	0.650	0.591	0.542	0.500	0.464	0.433	0.406	0.382	0.361	0.342	0.325	0.310	0.295
70	0.875	0.778	0.700	0.636	0.583	0.538	0.500	0.467	0.438	0.412	0.389	0.368	0.350	0.333	0.318
75	0.938	0.833	0.750	0.682	0.625	0.577	0.536	0.500	0.469	0.441	0.417	0.395	0.375	0.357	0.341
80	1.000	0.889	0.800	0.727	0.667	0.615	0.571	0.533	0.500	0.471	0.444	0.421	0.400	0.381	0.364
85	1.063	0.944	0.850	0.773	0.708	0.654	0.607	0.567	0.531	0.500	0.472	0.447	0.425	0.405	0.386
90	1.125	1.000	0.900	0.818	0.750	0.692	0.643	0.600	0.563	0.529	0.500	0.474	0.450	0.429	0.409
95	1.188	1.056	0.950	0.864	0.792	0.731	0.679	0.633	0.594	0.559	0.528	0.500	0.475	0.452	0.432
100	1.250	1.111	1.000	0.909	0.833	0.769	0.714	0.667	0.625	0.588	0.556	0.526	0.500	0.476	0.455
105	1.313	1.167	1.050	0.955	0.875	0.808	0.750	0.700	0.656	0.618	0.583	0.553	0.525	0.500	0.477
110	1.375	1.222	1.100	1.000	0.917	0.846	0.786	0.733	0.688	0.647	0.611	0.579	0.550	0.524	0.500
115	1.438	1.278	1.150	1.045	0.958	0.885	0.821	0.767	0.719	0.676	0.639	0.605	0.575	0.548	0.523
120	1.500	1.333	1.200	1.091	1.000	0.923	0.857	0.800	0.750	0.706	0.667	0.632	0.600	0.571	0.545

DRUG DOSE in mg/kg/hr

Patient's Weight kg / lbs	40 / 88	45 / 99	50 / 110	55 / 121	60 / 132	65 / 143	70 / 154	75 / 165	80 / 176	85 / 187	90 / 198	95 / 209	100 / 220	105 / 231	110 / 242
Infusion Rate in mL/hr															
5	0.12	0.11	0.10	0.09	0.08	0.08	0.07	0.07	0.06	0.06	0.06	0.05	0.05	0.05	0.05
10	0.25	0.22	0.20	0.18	0.17	0.15	0.14	0.13	0.12	0.12	0.11	0.11	0.10	0.10	0.09
15	0.37	0.33	0.30	0.27	0.25	0.23	0.21	0.20	0.19	0.18	0.17	0.16	0.15	0.14	0.14
20	0.50	0.44	0.40	0.36	0.33	0.31	0.29	0.27	0.25	0.24	0.22	0.21	0.20	0.19	0.18
25	0.62	0.56	0.50	0.45	0.42	0.38	0.36	0.33	0.31	0.29	0.28	0.26	0.25	1.24	0.23
30	0.75	0.67	0.60	0.55	0.50	0.46	0.43	0.40	0.37	0.35	0.33	0.32	0.30	0.29	0.27
35	0.87	0.78	0.70	0.64	0.58	0.54	0.50	0.47	0.44	0.41	0.39	0.37	0.35	0.33	0.32
40	1.00	0.89	0.80	0.73	0.67	0.62	0.57	0.53	0.50	0.47	0.44	0.42	0.40	0.38	0.36
45	1.13	1.00	0.90	0.82	0.75	0.69	0.64	0.60	0.56	0.53	0.50	0.47	0.45	0.43	0.41
50	1.25	1.11	1.00	0.91	0.83	0.77	0.71	0.67	0.62	0.59	0.56	0.53	0.50	0.48	0.45
55	1.38	1.22	1.10	1.00	0.92	0.85	0.79	0.73	0.69	0.65	0.61	0.58	0.55	0.52	0.50
60	1.50	1.33	1.20	1.09	1.00	0.92	0.86	0.80	0.75	0.71	0.67	0.63	0.60	0.57	0.55
65	1.63	1.44	1.30	1.18	1.08	1.00	0.93	0.87	0.81	0.76	0.72	0.68	0.65	0.62	0.59
70	1.75	1.56	1.40	1.27	1.17	1.08	1.00	0.93	0.87	0.82	0.78	0.74	0.70	0.67	0.64
75	1.87	1.67	1.50	1.36	1.25	1.15	1.07	1.00	0.94	0.88	0.83	0.79	0.75	0.71	0.68
80	2.00	1.78	1.60	1.45	1.33	1.23	1.14	1.07	1.00	0.94	0.89	0.84	0.80	0.76	0.73
85	2.13	1.89	1.70	1.55	0.42	1.31	1.21	1.13	1.06	1.00	0.94	0.89	0.85	0.81	0.77
90	2.25	2.00	1.80	1.64	1.50	1.38	1.29	1.20	1.13	1.06	1.00	0.95	0.90	0.86	0.82
95	2.38	2.11	1.90	1.73	1.58	1.46	1.36	1.27	1.19	1.12	1.06	1.00	0.95	0.90	0.86
100	2.50	2.22	2.00	1.82	1.67	1.54	1.43	1.33	1.25	1.18	1.11	1.05	1.00	0.95	0.91
105	2.63	2.33	2.10	1.91	1.75	1.62	1.50	1.40	1.31	1.24	1.17	1.11	1.05	1.00	0.95
110	2.75	2.44	2.20	2.00	1.83	1.69	1.57	1.47	1.38	1.29	1.22	1.16	1.10	1.05	1.00
115	2.88	2.56	2.30	2.09	1.92	1.77	1.64	1.53	1.44	1.35	1.28	1.21	1.15	1.10	1.05
120	3.00	2.67	2.40	2.18	2.00	1.85	1.71	1.60	1.50	1.41	1.33	1.26	1.20	1.14	1.09

Tissue-Type Plasminogen Activator (Alteplase) (Activase)

Pharmacology

Thrombolytic enzyme derived from either human melanoma cell culture (commercially available single chain t-PA) or recombinant DNA technology (double-chain rt-PA). The latter preparation is not commercially available

Single-chain alteplase has a higher clearance rate and reduced fibrinogenolytic activity than double-chain rt-PA. Physiologic and pharmacologic effects of exogenous t-PA preparations are similar to endogenous t-PA derived principally from vascular endothelium

Mechanism of action involves conversion of plasminogen to plasmin via peptide bond cleavage, thereby promoting degradation of fibrin, fibrinogen, and other plasma procoagulation proteins (factors V, VIII, XII)

Site of action is principally plasminogen found within the thrombus or embolus and not circulating plasminogen. This fibrin selectively may diminish

(continued below)

Administrative Guidelines

Administer infusion via precision control device

Continuously monitor ECG and carefully follow vital signs during infusion

When preparing infusions, do not add other medications to the vial and reconstitute only with sterile water for injection without preservatives. Do not dilute below a concentration of 0.5 mg/mL. Gently tilt and roll vial, but avoid shaking. Avoid using in-line filters owing to drug affinity for filter material and discard vial if vacuum is not present

Determine hematocrit, platelet count, prothrombin time, activated partial thromboplastin time, and cardiac enzymes, if possible, before use. Hemostatic indices are not essential in following lytic function

Vessel patency rates and mortality appear to be time dependent; therefore, earliest application feasible is recommended

(continued below)

development of a systemic lytic state and elaboration of significant fibrin degradation products

Thrombolytic efficacy may be less dependent on thrombus age than that observed with either urokinase or streptokinase

Fibrinolytic activity is highly variable between individuals but is more prolonged and intense than that observed with streptokinase

Effects of alteplase may be antagonized by plasminogen activating inhibitors (which are inversely related to thrombin levels) and circulating antiplasmins (alpha$_2$-antiplasmin, alpha$_2$-macroglobulin, antithrombin III and alpha$_1$-antitrypsin)

May produce additional anticoagulant effects by generating fibrinogen and fibrin degradation products and altering platelet function

Rethrombosis may occur by activation of plasminogen in vascular endothelium or platelets

C1 complement complexes and activation of the complement cascade may occur

(continued on page 290)

Avoid intramuscular injections before, during, and 24 hours after alteplase therapy. Do not attempt central venous access or arterial puncture during this period unless absolutely essential (upper extremity sites are preferred)

Minimize performance of venipuncture and handling of patient. Compress venipuncture sites for up to 30 minutes to control minor bleeding, apply a pressure dressing, and check the site frequently

Apply local pressure to minor surface bleeding areas as necessary but do ***not*** alter the infusion dose with superficial bleeding. Immediately discontinue therapy, however, if serious external or internal hemorrhage is observed

Efficacy and bleeding risk do not directly correlate with laboratory parameters of the lytic state

Contraindicated in those with known hypersensitivity, active internal bleeding or established bleeding diathesis, severe uncontrolled hypertension, intracranial tumor, aneurysm or arteriovenous

(continued on page 290)

Tissue-Type Plasminogen Activator (Alteplase) (Activase)

Activity is standardized and expressed in International Units (IU) based on in vitro clot lysis. Each milligram of commercially prepared alteplase is equivalent to 580,000 IU

Indications

Acute evolving transmural myocardial infarction—initiate therapy as soon as feasible and preferably ***within 6 hours*** of symptom onset. Patency rates and mortality may be both dose and time dependent

Acute massive ***diagnostically confirmed*** pulmonary embolism involving obstruction of at least one lobar artery or associated with unstable hemodynamics ***(employing intravenous infusion)***

Unlabeled Uses. Lysis by intra-arterial infusion of arterial emboli and thrombi involving cerebral, coronary, mesenteric, femoropopliteal, and basilar artery sites; pulmonary artery or rapid IV infusion for significant pulmonary emboli; intravenous clot dissolution of subclavian and deep vein thrombosis

malformation, intracranial or intraspinal surgery or trauma within 2 months, and history of a cerebrovascular accident

Use with extreme caution in patients with hypertension exceeding 180 mmHg systolic or 110 mmHg diastolic pressure and recent (within 10 days) serious trauma, major surgery, organ biopsy, gastrointestinal bleeding, obstetrical delivery, or puncture of a noncompressible artery

Use with caution in patients following cardiopulmonary resuscitation or minor trauma (within 10 days); in patients with suspected mural thrombus, pregnancy, hemorrhagic diabetic retinopathy, cerebrovascular disease, acute pericarditis, subacute bacterial endocarditis, septic thrombophlebitis or occluded arteriovenous cannula at the site of serious infection, severe hepatic or renal disease, or atrial fibrillation; in conditions associated with increased bleeding risk; and in those over 75 years of age

(continued below)

Pharmacokinetics

Onset of Action. Within 90 minutes

Peak Effects. Not specified by manufacturer

Duration of Action. Perhaps as long as 7 hours

Plasma (Distribution) Half-Life. 3.6–4.6 minutes

Tissue (Elimination) Half-Life. 39–53 minutes

Metabolism. Primarily via the liver

Overdosage may manifest with severe hemorrhage. Provide general supportive measures and fluid resuscitate with volume expanders other than dextran. Transfuse with packed red blood cells, fresh frozen plasma, and cryoprecipitate as needed. Although unproven, IV aminocaproic acid may be efficacious in life-threatening cases

...ype Plasminogen Activator (Alteplase) (Activase)

Dosing Information

Acute Myocardial Infarction

Standard Dosing Regimen. For patients weighing 65 kg or greater: Administer 100 mg IV over 3 hours as follows:

First hour	10 mg IV bolus over 1–2 minutes, then 50 mg IV infusion
Second hour	20 mg IV infusion over 60 minutes
Third hour	20 mg IV infusion over 60 minutes

For patients weighing less than 65 kg: Administer 1.25 mg/kg total dose over 3 hours as follows (do not exceed 100 mg total dose):

First hour	60% of total dose; 6–10 mg IV bolus, then remainder of 60% of dose infused over 60 minutes
Second hour	20% of total dose infused over 60 minutes
Third hour	20% of total dose infused over 60 minutes

(continued below)

Potential Drug Interactions

Potentiation of Alteplase Effects. Heparin, aspirin, oral anticoagulants, single-chain urokinase, dipyridamole, ticlopidine

Antagonism of Alteplase Effects. Aminocaproic acid

Principal Adverse Effects

CNS. Cerebrovascular hemorrhage and infarction

CV. Bradycardia and reperfusion-related atrial and ventricular dysrhythmias, hypotension

Heme. Spontaneous superficial and internal bleeding, unexplained thrombocytopenia

Allergic. Nausea, vomiting, fever, possible anaphylaxis, urticaria

Miscellaneous. Atheroemboli syndromes

Accelerated (GUSTO) Regimen. 15-mg IV bolus, then 0.75 mg/kg IV infusion over 30 minutes (not to exceed 50 mg), then 0.5 mg/kg IV infusion over 60 minutes (not to exceed 35 mg). Total dose administered should ***not*** exceed 100 mg

Pulmonary Emboli

100 mg IV infusion over 2 hours. Although unproven, 30–50 mg has been given directly into the pulmonary artery over 1.5–2.0 hours

Arterial Embolism or Thrombosis

0.02–0.1 mg/kg/hr ***intra-arterial*** infusion for 1–8 hours

To prevent recurrent emboli or thrombosis, heparin infusion ***preceded*** by a loading dose is recommended concomitant with alteplase therapy

How Supplied

1[illegible] mg/mL—20-mg vacuum vial (11.6 million IU) with [illegible] sterile water for injection as diluent
[illegible] 50-mg vacuum vial (29.0 million IU) with [illegible] water for injection as diluent
[illegible] vacuum vial (58.0 million IU) with [illegible] injection as diluent

…aphan Camsylate (Arfonad)

Pharmacology

Nondepolarizing ganglionic blocking agent, which stabilizes postsynaptic membranes against acetylcholine released from presynaptic nerve endings

Impedes transmission of impulses at both sympathetic and parasympathetic ganglia by competing with acetylcholine for autonomic cholinergic receptors

Produces peripheral vasodilation and decreased blood pressure by direct effects and blockade of sympathetic ganglia

Reduces cerebral, splanchnic, and renal blood flow—variable effects on cardiac output and heart rate

Parasympathetic blockade may precipitate atony of the bladder and gastrointestinal tract, xerostomia, anhidrosis, mydriasis, and cycloplegia

May release histamine

Tachyphylaxis can occur after 24–72 hours

Administrative Guidelines

Administer infusion via precision control device

Continuously monitor blood pressure and ECG—carefully observe respiratory status because apnea has occurred

Insure adequate oxygenation during use

Always dilute before use—recommend 5% dextrose injection USP

Do not admix infusion solution with other drugs—incompatible with thiopental, alkaline solutions, bromides, iodides, tubocurarine chloride, and gallamine triethiodide

Pupillary dilation does ***not*** reflect depth of anesthesia or anoxia

Initiate oral antihypertensive therapy as soon as feasible before tachyphylaxis develops

(continued below)

Indications

Short-term control of blood pressure during surgery, hypertensive emergencies, and pulmonary edema associated with pulmonary and systemic hypertension

Unlabeled Uses. Blood pressure control in acute aortic dissection and ischemic heart disease

Pharmacokinetics

Onset of Action. Almost immediately

Peak Effects. Approximately 5 minutes

Duration of Action. 10–30 minutes

Metabolism. Via pseudocholinesterase with renal filtration and secretion

Contraindicated in patients with uncorrected anemia or respiratory insufficiency, shock, hypovolemia, and asphyxia. Glaucoma and inability to replace fluids and blood may also be contraindications

Use with caution in elderly or debilitated patients; those with hypotension or hypovolemia; renal, hepatic, or pulmonary disease; CNS disease; Addison's disease; diabetes; history of allergy; arteriosclerotic cardiovascular disease; and those on corticosteroids or antihypertensive medications

Overdosage typically produces excessive hypotension. Manage by terminating infusion, providing supportive measures, and assisting patient to the Trendelenburg position. Consider phenylephrine initially for severe cases and norepinephrine for refractory hypotension

Trimethaphan Camsylate (Arfonad)

Dosing Information

Initial Infusion Rate. 0.5–4 mg/min

Maintenance Infusion Range. 0.3–6.0 mg/min

Maximum Infusion Rate. Rarely greater than 6 mg/min

Titration Guideline

Suggested Regimen. Adjust infusion by 0.5–1.0 mg/min every 5–10 minutes as necessary

How Supplied

50 mg/mL—10-mL ampuls of 500 mg

Potential Drug Interactions

Potentiation of Trimethaphan Effects. Procainamide, halothane, spinal anesthetics, diuretics, antihypertensive agents

Possibly Potentiated by Trimethaphan. Tubocurarine or succinylcholine chloride and neuromuscular blocking drugs

Principal Adverse Effects

CNS. Restlessness, weakness, cycloplegia, mydriasis

Pulmonary. Apnea, respiratory arrest

CV. Hypotension, tachycardia, and angina

GI. Nausea, vomiting, anorexia, dry mouth

GU. Urinary retention

Allergic. Urticaria, pruritus

Miscellaneous. Elevation of glucose and decrease of serum potassium

Trimethaphan Camsylate (Arfonad) 1500 mg in 500 mL

■ Infusion Rate in mL/hr (pump setting) ■ Drug Dose in mg/min

mL/hr	mg/min	mL/hr	mg/min	mL/hr	mg/min	mL/hr	mg/min	mL/hr	mg/min	mL/hr	mg/min
1	0.05	21	1.05	41	2.05	61	3.05	81	4.05	101	5.05
2	0.10	22	1.10	42	2.10	62	3.10	82	4.10	102	5.10
3	0.15	23	1.15	43	2.15	63	3.15	83	4.15	103	5.15
4	0.20	24	1.20	44	2.20	64	3.20	84	4.20	104	5.20
5	0.25	25	1.25	45	2.25	65	3.25	85	4.25	105	5.25
6	0.30	26	1.30	46	2.30	66	3.30	86	4.30	106	5.30
7	0.35	27	1.35	47	2.35	67	3.35	87	4.35	107	5.35
8	0.40	28	1.40	48	2.40	68	3.40	88	4.40	108	5.40
9	0.45	29	1.45	49	2.45	69	3.45	89	4.45	109	5.45
10	0.50	30	1.50	50	2.50	70	3.50	90	4.50	110	5.50
11	0.55	31	1.55	51	2.55	71	3.55	91	4.55	111	5.55
12	0.60	32	1.60	52	2.60	72	3.60	92	4.60	112	5.60
13	0.65	33	1.65	53	2.65	73	3.65	93	4.65	113	5.65
14	0.70	34	1.70	54	2.70	74	3.70	94	4.70	114	5.70
15	0.75	35	1.75	55	2.75	75	3.75	95	4.75	115	5.75
16	0.80	36	1.80	56	2.80	76	3.80	96	4.80	116	5.80
17	0.85	37	1.85	57	2.85	77	3.85	97	4.85	117	5.85
18	0.90	38	1.90	58	2.90	78	3.90	98	4.90	118	5.90
19	0.95	39	1.95	59	2.95	79	3.95	99	4.95	119	5.95
20	1.00	40	2.00	60	3.00	80	4.00	100	5.00	120	6.00

■ Infusion Rate in mL/hr (pump setting) ■ Drug Dose in mg/min

Infusion Rate	Drug Dose	Infusion Rate	Drug Dose	Infusion Rate	Drug Dose	Infusion Rate	Drug Dose	Infusion Rate	Drug Dose	Infusion Rate	Drug Dose
1	0.10	21	2.10	41	4.10	61	6.10	81	8.10	101	10.10
2	0.20	22	2.20	42	4.20	62	6.20	82	8.20	102	10.20
3	0.30	23	2.30	43	4.30	63	6.30	83	8.30	103	10.30
4	0.40	24	2.40	44	4.40	64	6.40	84	8.40	104	10.40
5	0.50	25	2.50	45	4.50	65	6.50	85	8.50	105	10.50
6	0.60	26	2.60	46	4.60	66	6.60	86	8.60	106	10.60
7	0.70	27	2.70	47	4.70	67	6.70	87	8.70	107	10.70
8	0.80	28	2.80	48	4.80	68	6.80	88	8.80	108	10.80
9	0.90	29	2.90	49	4.90	69	6.90	89	8.90	109	10.90
10	1.00	30	3.00	50	5.00	70	7.00	90	9.00	110	11.00
11	1.10	31	3.10	51	5.10	71	7.10	91	9.10	111	11.10
12	1.20	32	3.20	52	5.20	72	7.20	92	9.20	112	11.20
13	1.30	33	3.30	53	5.30	73	7.30	93	9.30	113	11.30
14	1.40	34	3.40	54	5.40	74	7.40	94	9.40	114	11.40
15	1.50	35	3.50	55	5.50	75	7.50	95	9.50	115	11.50
16	1.60	36	3.60	56	5.60	76	7.60	96	9.60	116	11.60
17	1.70	37	3.70	57	5.70	77	7.70	97	9.70	117	11.70
18	1.80	38	3.80	58	5.80	78	7.80	98	9.80	118	11.80
19	1.90	39	3.90	59	5.90	79	7.90	99	9.90	119	11.90
20	2.00	40	4.00	60	6.00	80	8.00	100	10.00	120	12.00

Urokinase (Abbokinase)

Pharmacology

Thrombolytic enzyme derived from human kidney tissue cultures

Mechanism of action involves conversion of plasminogen to plasmin via peptide bond cleavage, thereby promoting degradation of fibrin, fibrinogen, and other plasma procoagulant proteins (factors V, VIII, XII)

Site of action includes plasminogen found on the surface and within thrombi and emboli. Also activates circulating plasminogen and contributes to a systemic lytic state

May produce additional anticoagulant effects by generating high levels of fibrin and fibrinogen degradation products

Activity standardized and expressed in International Units (IU) based on in vitro ability to lyse fibrin clot

Administrative Guidelines

Administer infusion via precision control device

Continuously monitor ECG and carefully follow vital signs during infusion

When preparing infusion, reconstitute immediately before use only with sterile water for injection without preservatives—gently tilt and roll vial but do not shake

Do not use if highly colored or heavy concentration of filaments is noted

Obtain thrombin, prothrombin, and activated partial thromboplastin times and hemoglobin, hematocrit, and platelet counts, if possible, before initiating therapy. Consider thrombin times every 4 hours during treatment to assess lytic state

Do not begin urokinase in cases of a suspected bleeding diathesis unless the thrombin time is less than twice the control value

(continued below)

Indications

Acute (within 5 days), massive ***diagnostically confirmed*** pulmonary emboli involving at least two lobar arteries (or equivalent clot burden in other pulmonary vessels) or associated with unstable hemodynamics

Intracoronary administration within 6 hours of evolving acute transmural myocardial infarction

Lysis of obstructed intravenous catheters occluded only by clotted blood or fibrin

Unlabeled Uses. Intravenous administration for acute myocardial infarction; lysis of arteriovenous cannulae; clot dissolution with retinal vessel occlusion and varied thromboembolic disorders, including angiographically confirmed coronary thrombi

(continued on page 302)

Avoid intramuscular injections before, during, and 24 hours after urokinase therapy. Do not attempt central venous access or arterial puncture during this period unless absolutely essential (upper extremity sites are recommended)

Minimize performance of venipuncture and handling of patient. Compress venipuncture sites for up to 30 minutes to control minor bleeding, apply a pressure dressing, and check the site frequently

Apply local pressure to minor surface bleeding areas as necessary, but do ***not*** alter the infusion dose with superficial bleeding. Immediately discontinue therapy, however, if serious external or internal hemorrhage is observed

Efficacy and bleeding risk do not directly correlate with laboratory parameters of the lytic state

Contraindicated with known hypersensitivity, active internal bleeding, severe uncontrolled hypertension, intracranial tumor, aneurysm or arteriovenous malformation, intracranial or intraspinal surgery or trauma, and cerebrovascular accident within 2 months

(continued on page 302)

Urokinase (Abbokinase)

Pharmacokinetics

Onset of Action. Within 15 minutes
Peak Effects. Not specified by manufacturer
Duration of Action. At least several hours
Plasma Half-Life. Approximately 10–20 minutes
Metabolism. Via liver

Use with extreme caution in patients with hypertension exceeding 180 mmHg systolic or 110 mmHg diastolic pressure and recent (within 10 days) serious trauma, major surgery, organ biopsy, gastrointestinal bleeding, obstetrical delivery, or puncture of a noncompressible artery

Use with caution in patients following cardiopulmonary resuscitation, or minor trauma within 10 days; in those with suspected mural thrombus, pregnancy, hemorrhagic diabetic retinopathy, cerebrovascular disease, acute pericarditis, subacute bacterial endocarditis, septic thrombophlebitis or occluded arteriovenous cannula at the site of serious infection, severe hepatic or renal disease, or atrial fibrillation; in conditions associated with increased bleeding risk; and in those over 75 years of age

Overdosage may manifest with severe hemorrhage. Provide general supportive measures and fluid resuscitate with volume expanders other than dextran. Transfuse with packed red blood cells, fresh frozen plasma, and cryoprecipitate as needed. Although unproven, IV aminocaproic acid may be efficacious in life-threatening cases

Dosing Information

Pulmonary Embolism

4400 units/kg IV bolus over 10 minutes. Then 4400 units/kg/hr infusion for 12 hours. To prevent recurrent emboli, initiate heparin infusion ***without*** a loading dose ***after*** the thrombin time has decreased to less than twice the control value (generally 3–4 hours after termination of urokinase infusion)

Acute Myocardial Infarction

Intracoronary Regimen. 6000 units/min for up to 2 hours and until artery is maximally opened. Administer 2500–10,000 units IV heparin bolus ***before*** urokinase use, and subsequently initiate a heparin infusion. Approximately 500,000 units total dose for urokinase is usually required for coronary thrombolysis

Intravenous Regimen. 1–1.5 million units IV bolus over 5 minutes, then 1–1.5 million units infusion over 45–90 minutes. Administer 5000-unit heparin bolus concomitantly with or immediately after the urokinase infusion (2–3 million units of urokinase has alternatively been given as an IV bolus dose over 5 minutes)

(continued on page 304)

Potential Drug Interactions

Potentiation of Urokinase Effects. Heparin, oral anticoagulants, aspirin, dipyridamole, indomethacin, phenylbutazone, sulfinpyrazone, ticlopidine

Antagonism of Urokinase Effects. Aminocaproic acid

Principal Adverse Effects

CNS. Cerebrovascular hemorrhage, rigors

CV. Reperfusion-related atrial and ventricular dysrhythmias

Heme. Spontaneous superficial and internal bleeding, unexplained decrease in hematocrit

Allergic. Rash, bronchospasm, and possible anaphylaxis

Miscellaneous. Fever

Urokinase (Abbokinase)

Intracoronary Thrombi Lysis

Suggest 500,000–750,000 units intracoronary bolus over 5 minutes, then 100,000 units/hr for up to 24–48 hours. Periodic angiographic revisualization of the coronary artery is recommended

Occluded Catheters

5000 units gently injected into the catheter employing a tuberculin syringe. Avoid excessive pressure. Aseptically attempt aspiration of clotted catheter with 5-mL syringe after 5 minutes. May repeat aspiration every 5 minutes up to 30 minutes. Consider repeat 5000-unit urokinase dose in refractory cases after additional 30 minutes of observation. Once patency is achieved, aspirate 4–5 mL of blood to insure removal of all particulate debris and residual drug

How Supplied

IV Catheter Clearance. 5000 units/mL—1-mL univials of 5000 units

Parenteral Injection. 250,000 units/mL—5-mL vials of 1,250,000 units

Urokinase (Abbokinase) 1,250,000 units in 250 mL

■ **Infusion Rate in mL/hr (pump setting)** ■ **Drug Dose in units/hr**

mL/hr	units/hr	mL/hr	units/hr	mL/hr	units/hr	mL/hr	units/hr	mL/hr	units/hr	mL/hr	units/hr
1	5,000	21	105,000	41	205,000	61	305,000	81	405,000	101	505,000
2	10,000	22	110,000	42	210,000	62	310,000	82	410,000	102	510,000
3	15,000	23	115,000	43	215,000	63	315,000	83	415,000	103	515,000
4	20,000	24	120,000	44	220,000	64	320,000	84	420,000	104	520,000
5	25,000	25	125,000	45	225,000	65	325,000	85	425,000	105	525,000
6	30,000	26	130,000	46	230,000	66	330,000	86	430,000	106	530,000
7	35,000	27	135,000	47	235,000	67	335,000	87	435,000	107	535,000
8	40,000	28	140,000	48	240,000	68	340,000	88	440,000	108	540,000
9	45,000	29	145,000	49	245,000	69	345,000	89	445,000	109	545,000
10	50,000	30	150,000	50	250,000	70	350,000	90	450,000	110	550,000
11	55,000	31	155,000	51	255,000	71	355,000	91	455,000	111	555,000
12	60,000	32	160,000	52	260,000	72	360,000	92	460,000	112	560,000
13	65,000	33	165,000	53	265,000	73	365,000	93	465,000	113	565,000
14	70,000	34	170,000	54	270,000	74	370,000	94	470,000	114	570,000
15	75,000	35	175,000	55	275,000	75	375,000	95	475,000	115	575,000
16	80,000	36	180,000	56	280,000	76	380,000	96	480,000	116	580,000
17	85,000	37	185,000	57	285,000	77	385,000	97	485,000	117	585,000
18	90,000	38	190,000	58	290,000	78	390,000	98	490,000	118	590,000
19	95,000	39	195,000	59	295,000	79	395,000	99	495,000	119	595,000
20	100,000	40	200,000	60	300,000	80	400,000	100	500,000	120	600,000

DRUG DOSE in units/kg/hr

Infusion Rate in mL/hr	Patient's Weight kg / lbs: 40 / 88	45 / 99	50 / 110	55 / 121	60 / 132	65 / 143	70 / 154	75 / 165	80 / 176	85 / 187	90 / 198	95 / 209	100 / 220	105 / 231	110 / 242
5	625	556	500	455	417	385	357	333	313	294	278	263	250	238	227
10	1,250	1,111	1,000	909	833	769	714	667	625	588	556	526	500	476	455
15	1,875	1,667	1,500	1,364	1,250	1,154	1,071	1,000	938	882	833	789	750	714	682
20	2,500	2,222	2,000	1,818	1,667	1,538	1,429	1,333	1,250	1,176	1,111	1,053	1,000	952	909
25	3,125	2,778	2,500	2,273	2,083	1,923	1,786	1,667	1,563	1,471	1,389	1,316	1,250	1,190	1,136
30	3,750	3,333	3,000	2,727	2,500	2,308	2,143	2,000	1,875	1,765	1,667	1,579	1,500	1,429	1,364
35	4,375	3,889	3,500	3,182	2,917	2,692	2,500	2,333	2,188	2,059	1,944	1,842	1,750	1,667	1,591
40	5,000	4,444	4,000	3,636	3,333	3,077	2,857	2,667	2,500	2,353	2,222	2,105	2,000	1,905	1,818
45	5,625	5,000	4,500	4,091	3,750	3,462	3,214	3,000	2,813	2,647	2,500	2,368	2,250	2,143	2,045
50	6,250	5,556	5,000	4,545	4,167	3,846	3,571	3,333	3,125	2,941	2,778	2,632	2,500	2,381	2,273
55	6,875	6,111	5,500	5,000	4,583	4,231	3,929	3,667	3,438	3,235	3,056	2,895	2,750	2,619	2,500
60	7,500	6,667	6,000	5,455	5,000	4,615	4,286	4,000	3,750	3,529	3,333	3,158	3,000	2,857	2,727
65	8,125	7,222	6,500	5,909	5,417	5,000	4,643	4,333	4,063	3,824	3,611	3,421	3,250	3,095	2,955
70	8,750	7,778	7,000	6,364	5,833	5,385	5,000	4,667	4,375	4,118	3,889	3,684	3,500	3,333	3,182
75	9,375	8,333	7,500	6,818	6,250	5,769	5,357	5,000	4,688	4,412	4,167	3,947	3,750	3,571	3,409
80	10,000	8,889	8,000	7,273	6,667	6,154	5,714	5,333	5,000	4,706	4,444	4,211	4,000	3,810	3,636
85	10,625	9,444	8,500	7,727	7,083	6,538	6,071	5,667	5,313	5,000	4,722	4,474	4,250	4,048	3,864
90	11,250	10,000	9,000	8,182	7,500	6,923	6,429	6,000	5,625	5,294	5,000	4,737	4,500	4,286	4,091
95	11,875	10,556	9,500	8,636	7,917	7,308	6,786	6,333	5,938	5,588	5,278	5,000	4,750	4,524	4,318
100	12,500	11,111	10,000	9,091	8,333	7,692	7,143	6,667	6,250	5,882	5,556	5,263	5,000	4,762	4,545
105	13,125	11,667	10,500	9,545	8,750	8,077	7,500	7,000	6,563	6,176	5,833	5,526	5,250	5,000	4,773
110	13,750	12,222	11,000	10,000	9,167	8,462	7,857	7,333	6,875	6,471	6,111	5,789	5,500	5,238	5,000
115	14,375	12,778	11,500	10,455	9,583	8,846	8,214	7,667	7,188	6,765	6,389	6,053	5,750	5,476	5,227
120	15,000	13,333	12,000	10,909	10,000	9,231	8,571	8,000	7,500	7,059	6,667	6,316	6,000	5,714	5,455

Vasopressin (Pitressin)

Pharmacology

Endogenous arginine polypeptide stored in the posterior pituitary following hypothalamic neuronal secretion

Primary mechanism of action involves activation of adenyl cyclase in the renal tubules, thereby increasing cyclic adenosine monophosphate. This, in turn, promotes water and urea conservation and an antidiuretic effect as well as preserving serum osmolality

Smooth muscle vasoconstrictor at the capillary and arteriolar levels with reduced blood flow to skin, splanchnic, gastrointestinal, coronary, and muscular beds

Intra-arterial celiac infusion constricts all major arterial branches except the hepatic artery and lowers portal venous pressure

May decrease heart rate and cardiac output and precipitate acute myocardial infarction—pulmonary and systemic blood pressures may increase

(continued below)

Administrative Guidelines

Administer infusion via precision control device

Carefully monitor ECG and vital signs—closely follow hematologic parameters and electrolytes and fluid balance

Administer via central line, if possible, or large vein. May infuse selectively intra-arterially, especially when IV therapy is ineffective (usually into the superior mesenteric artery)

Carefully observe IV infusion site for free flow, blanching, and extravasation

Extravasation requires immediate discontinuation of infusion; consider subcutaneous infiltration of 5–10 mg phentolamine mesylate in 10–15 mL saline

Attempt to taper infusion after 24 hours, if clinically acceptable, but may administer for 3–14 days

Contraindicated in those with known hypersensitivity or chronic nephritis associated with significant nitrogen retention

(continued below)

Increases peristaltic activity, especially in the large intestine; gastrointestinal sphincter tone; and gallbladder and urinary bladder contraction

Facilitates release of growth hormone, follicle-stimulating hormone, and corticotropin

Potency standardized based on pressor response in rats and expressed in USP units

Indications

Replacement therapy of antidiuretic hormone in neurogenic diabetes insipidus; stimulation of peristalsis with abdominal distention and intestinal paresis; adjunct to abdominal roentgenography and renal biopsy to dispel overlying gas shadows

Unlabeled Uses. Intravenous and intra-arterial infusion to prevent and control significant gastrointestinal hemorrhage; provocative test for assessment of pituitary release of growth hormone and corticotropin

Use with caution in patients with asthma, seizures, migraine, heart failure, coronary heart disease, renal disease, arteriosclerosis, goiter with cardiac involvement, or conditions in which extracellular volume expansion may be detrimental

Overdosage may manifest with signs of water intoxication, including headache, confusion, drowsiness, anuria, weight gain, seizures, and coma. Restrict free water; discontinue infusion; and consider mannitol, hypertonic dextrose, urea, and furosemide. A urine specific gravity of less than 1.015 and polyuria are desirable

Vasopressin (Pitressin)

Pharmacokinetics

Onset of Action. 30–60 minutes

Peak Effects. Within 1–2 hours

Duration of Action. 1–2 hours

Plasma (Distribution) Half-Life. 10–20 minutes

Metabolism. Via liver and kidneys

Dosing Information

Initial Infusion Rate. 0.2–0.4 units/min IV; 0.1–0.5 units/min intra-arterial

Maintenance Infusion Range. 0.1–0.9 units/min

Maximum Infusion Rate. 0.9 units/min

Titration Guideline

Suggested Regimen. Adjust infusion by 0.1 unit/min every 30–60 minutes as necessary for bleeding control

How Supplied

20 units/mL—0.5-mL ampuls of 10 units
1.0-mL ampuls of 20 units

Potential Drug Interactions

Potentiation of Vasopressin Effects. Chlorpropamide, clofibrate, carbamazepine, urea, phenformin, tricyclic antidepressants, fluorocortisone, ganglionic blockers
Antagonism of Vasopressin Effects. Lithium, epinephrine, alcohol, heparin, demeclocycline

Principal Adverse Effects

CNS. Circumoral pallor, tremor, vertigo, headache, diaphoresis, listlessness, confusion, lethargy, seizures, and coma
CV. Hypertension, cardiac arrest, angina, myocardial infarction, bradycardia, heart block, atrial dysrhythmias, peripheral vasoconstriction, and vascular collapse
GI. Nausea, vomiting, flatus, diarrhea, abdominal pain, ischemic colitis and bowel infarction, eructation
Dermatological. Sloughing and necrosis of skin at infusion site, cutaneous gangrene
Allergic. Anaphylaxis, urticaria, bronchial constriction, fever, angioedema, rash, wheezing, dyspnea, hypotension
Miscellaneous. Bilateral nipple necrosis

Vasopressin (Pitressin) 150 units in 250 mL

■ **Infusion Rate in mL/hr (pump setting)** ■ **Drug Dose in units/min**

mL/hr	units/min	mL/hr	units/min	mL/hr	units/min	mL/hr	units/min	mL/hr	units/min	mL/hr	units/min
1	0.01	21	0.21	41	0.41	61	0.61	81	0.81	101	1.01
2	0.02	22	0.22	42	0.42	62	0.62	82	0.82	102	1.02
3	0.03	23	0.23	43	0.43	63	0.63	83	0.83	103	1.03
4	0.04	24	0.24	44	0.44	64	0.64	84	0.84	104	1.04
5	0.05	25	0.25	45	0.45	65	0.65	85	0.85	105	1.05
6	0.06	26	0.26	46	0.46	66	0.66	86	0.86	106	1.06
7	0.07	27	0.27	47	0.47	67	0.67	87	0.87	107	1.07
8	0.08	28	0.28	48	0.48	68	0.68	88	0.88	108	1.08
9	0.09	29	0.29	49	0.49	69	0.69	89	0.89	109	1.09
10	0.10	30	0.30	50	0.50	70	0.70	90	0.90	110	1.10
11	0.11	31	0.31	51	0.51	71	0.71	91	0.91	111	1.11
12	0.12	32	0.32	52	0.52	72	0.72	92	0.92	112	1.12
13	0.13	33	0.33	53	0.53	73	0.73	93	0.93	113	1.13
14	0.14	34	0.34	54	0.54	74	0.74	94	0.94	114	1.14
15	0.15	35	0.35	55	0.55	75	0.75	95	0.95	115	1.15
16	0.16	36	0.36	56	0.56	76	0.76	96	0.96	116	1.16
17	0.17	37	0.37	57	0.57	77	0.77	97	0.97	117	1.17
18	0.18	38	0.38	58	0.58	78	0.78	98	0.98	118	1.18
19	0.19	39	0.39	59	0.59	79	0.79	99	0.99	119	1.19
20	0.20	40	0.40	60	0.60	80	0.80	100	1.00	120	1.20

Vasopressin (Pitressin) 250 units in 250 mL

■ Infusion Rate in mL/hr (pump setting) ■ Drug Dose in units/min

mL/hr	units/min	mL/hr	units/min	mL/hr	units/min	mL/hr	units/min	mL/hr	units/min	mL/hr	units/min
1	0.01	21	0.35	41	0.68	61	1.01	81	1.35	101	1.68
2	0.03	22	0.36	42	0.70	62	1.03	82	1.36	102	1.70
3	0.05	23	0.38	43	0.71	63	1.05	83	1.38	103	1.71
4	0.06	24	0.40	44	0.73	64	1.06	84	1.40	104	1.73
5	0.08	25	0.41	45	0.75	65	1.08	85	1.41	105	1.75
6	0.10	26	0.43	46	0.76	66	1.10	86	1.43	106	1.76
7	0.11	27	0.45	47	0.78	67	1.11	87	1.45	107	1.78
8	0.13	28	0.46	48	0.80	68	1.13	88	1.46	108	1.80
9	0.15	29	0.48	49	0.81	69	1.15	89	1.48	109	1.81
10	0.16	30	0.50	50	0.83	70	1.16	90	1.50	110	1.83
11	0.18	31	0.51	51	0.85	71	1.18	91	1.51	111	1.85
12	0.20	32	0.53	52	0.86	72	1.20	92	1.53	112	1.86
13	0.21	33	0.55	53	0.88	73	1.21	93	1.55	113	1.88
14	0.23	34	0.56	54	0.90	74	1.23	94	1.56	114	1.90
15	0.25	35	0.58	55	0.91	75	1.25	95	1.58	115	1.91
16	0.26	36	0.60	56	0.93	76	1.26	96	1.60	116	1.93
17	0.28	37	0.61	57	0.95	77	1.28	97	1.61	117	1.95
18	0.30	38	0.63	58	0.96	78	1.30	98	1.63	118	1.96
19	0.31	39	0.65	59	0.98	79	1.31	99	1.65	119	1.98
20	0.33	40	0.66	60	1.00	80	1.33	100	1.66	120	2.00

Vecuronium Bromide (Norcuron)

Pharmacology

Nondepolarizing neuromuscular blocking agent, which competes for cholinergic receptors at the motor end plate

Produces relatively short-acting skeletal muscle paralysis via reduced acetylcholine responsiveness at the myoneural junction

No significant effects on histamine release or cumulative effects

Minimal, if any, effects on cardiovascular system and blood pressure

No significant direct effects on cerebration, consciousness, or pain

Effects begin with eyes, face, and neck and then spread to limbs and trunk. Diaphragm is last affected. Recovery proceeds in the reverse order

Potency greater than pancuronium and atracurium

Administrative Guidelines

Administer infusion via precision control device

Continuously monitor ECG and vital signs

Do not administer through the same site with alkaline solutions or by intramuscular injections

Always have anticholinesterase reversal agents, endotracheal intubation equipment, mechanical ventilation, and skilled personnel in attendance

Use only after unconsciousness produced and adequate general anesthesia applied

Allow patients to recover from succinylcholine before use

Carefully monitor adductor pollicis muscle with twitch response to peripheral nerve stimulator

Observe for development of malignant hyperthermia and bradycardia

(continued below)

Indications

Skeletal muscle relaxation during surgery

Increase pulmonary compliance during mechanical ventilation after general anesthesia

Unlabeled Uses. Facilitation of mechanical ventilation in ICUs and endotracheal intubation

Pharmacokinetics

Onset of Action. Within 1 minute

Peak Effects. 3–5 minutes

Duration of Effects. 20–60 minutes

Distribution Half-Life. 3–14 minutes

Elimination Half-Life. 31–103 minutes

Metabolism. Not precisely defined but up to 50% may be eliminated in bile. Highly protein bound

Consider reduced dose in patients with severe renal and hepatic disease, neuromuscular disease, carcinomatosis, or severe electrolyte disorders

Tachyphylaxis may develop in burn patients

Contraindicated in patients with known hypersensitivity

Use with caution in those with hepatic dysfunction; obese patients; those with neuromuscular disease or electrolyte abnormalities; burn patients; renal and heart failure patients; and nursing women

Overdosage may potentiate pharmacologic effects, including profound weakness, respiratory depression, and apnea. Manage with appropriate fluids, cardiopulmonary supportive measures, and mechanical ventilation. Consider anticholinesterase agents such as neostigmine and anticholinergic drugs such as atropine. There is no established role for dialysis

Vecuronium Bromide (Norcuron)

Dosing Information

Initial Intubating Dose. 0.08–0.1 mg/kg IV bolus (80–100 μg/kg)

Initial Dose with General Anesthetics. 0.06–0.085 mg/kg (60–85 μg/kg)

Initial Dose with Succinylcholine. 0.005–0.06 mg/kg (5–60 μg/kg)

Initial Dose with Neuromuscular Diseases. 0.005–0.02 mg/kg (5–20 μg/kg)

Maintenance Intermittent IV Dose. 0.008–0.015 mg/kg (8–15 μg/kg)

Initial IV Infusion Dose. 0.001 mg/kg/min (1 μg/kg/min) begun 10–40 min after IV bolus dose given

Maintenance Infusion Rate. 0.8–1.2 μg/kg/min

Maximum Infusion Rate. 1.67 μg/kg/min

Potential Drug Interactions

Potentiation of Vecuronium Effects. Enflurane, isoflurane, halothane, cholinergic and cholinesterase drugs, acidosis, polymyxins, aminoglycosides, magnesium salts, quinidine, tetracycline, and succinylcholine

Antagonism of Vecuronium Effects. Alkalosis, anticholinesterase, and anticholinergic agents

Principal Adverse Effects

CNS. Muscle atrophy, weakness, and prolonged paralysis (especially in intensive care settings)

CV. Transient hypotension and tachycardia

Skin. Urticaria, rash, and injection site reaction

Allergic. Anaphylactoid and other histamine-mediated responses (rare)

Titration Guideline

Suggested Regimen. Adjust infusion by 0.1–0.2 μg/kg/min as necessary to achieve 90–95% neuromuscular blockade assessed by fast twitch response

How Supplied

1 mg/mL—10-mL vial of 10 mg

2 mg/mL—5-mL vial of 10 mg

Vecuronium Bromide (Norcuron) 100 mg in 500 mL

DRUG DOSE in µg/kg/min

Patient's Weight kg / lbs	40 / 88	45 / 99	50 / 110	55 / 121	60 / 132	65 / 143	70 / 154	75 / 165	80 / 176	85 / 187	90 / 198	95 / 209	100 / 220	105 / 231	110 / 242
Infusion Rate in mL/hr															
5	0.42	0.37	0.33	0.30	0.28	0.26	0.24	0.22	0.21	0.20	0.19	0.18	0.17	0.16	0.15
10	0.83	0.74	0.67	0.61	0.56	0.51	0.48	0.44	0.42	0.39	0.37	0.35	0.33	0.32	0.30
15	1.25	1.11	1.00	0.91	0.83	0.77	0.71	0.67	0.63	0.59	0.56	0.53	0.50	0.48	0.45
20	1.67	1.48	1.33	1.21	1.11	1.03	0.95	0.89	0.83	0.78	0.74	0.70	0.67	0.63	0.61
25	2.08	1.85	1.67	1.52	1.39	1.28	1.19	1.11	1.04	0.98	0.93	0.88	0.83	0.79	0.76
30	2.50	2.22	2.00	1.82	1.67	1.54	1.43	1.33	1.25	1.18	1.11	1.05	1.00	0.95	0.91
35	2.92	2.59	2.33	2.12	1.94	1.79	1.67	1.56	1.46	1.37	1.30	1.23	1.17	1.11	1.06
40	3.33	2.96	2.67	2.42	2.22	2.05	1.90	1.78	1.67	1.57	1.48	1.40	1.33	1.27	1.21
45	3.75	3.33	3.00	2.73	2.50	2.31	2.14	2.00	1.88	1.76	1.67	1.58	1.50	1.43	1.36
50	4.17	3.70	3.33	3.03	2.78	2.56	2.38	2.22	2.08	1.96	1.85	1.75	1.67	1.59	1.52
55	4.58	4.07	3.67	3.33	3.06	2.82	2.62	2.44	2.29	2.16	2.04	1.93	1.83	1.75	1.67
60	5.00	4.44	4.00	3.64	3.33	3.08	2.86	2.67	2.50	2.35	2.22	2.11	2.00	1.90	1.82
65	5.42	4.81	4.33	3.94	3.61	3.33	3.10	2.89	2.71	2.55	2.41	2.28	2.17	2.06	1.97
70	5.83	5.19	4.67	4.24	3.89	3.59	3.33	3.11	2.92	2.75	2.59	2.46	2.33	2.22	2.12
75	6.25	5.56	5.00	4.55	4.17	3.85	3.57	3.33	3.13	2.94	2.78	2.63	2.50	2.38	2.27
80	6.67	5.93	5.33	4.85	4.44	4.10	3.81	3.56	3.33	3.14	2.96	2.81	2.67	2.54	2.42
85	7.08	6.30	5.67	5.15	4.72	4.36	4.05	3.78	3.54	3.33	3.15	2.98	2.83	2.70	2.58
90	7.50	6.67	6.00	5.45	5.00	4.62	4.29	4.00	3.75	3.53	3.33	3.16	3.00	2.86	2.73
95	7.92	7.04	6.33	5.76	5.28	4.87	4.52	4.22	3.96	3.73	3.52	3.33	3.17	3.02	2.88
100	8.33	7.41	6.67	6.06	5.56	5.13	4.76	4.44	4.17	3.92	3.70	3.51	3.33	3.17	3.03
105	8.75	7.78	7.00	6.36	5.83	5.38	5.00	4.67	4.38	4.12	3.89	3.68	3.50	3.33	3.18
110	9.17	8.15	7.33	6.67	6.11	5.64	5.24	4.89	4.58	4.31	4.07	3.86	3.67	3.49	3.33
115	9.58	8.52	7.67	6.97	6.39	5.90	5.48	5.11	4.79	4.51	4.26	4.04	3.83	3.65	3.48
120	10.00	8.89	8.00	7.27	6.67	6.15	5.71	5.33	5.00	4.71	4.44	4.21	4.00	3.81	3.64

DRUG DOSE in μg/kg/min

Patient's Weight

Infusion Rate in mL/hr	kg / lbs: 40 / 88	45 / 99	50 / 110	55 / 121	60 / 132	65 / 143	70 / 154	75 / 165	80 / 176	85 / 187	90 / 198	95 / 209	100 / 220	105 / 231	110 / 242
5	0.83	0.74	0.66	0.60	0.55	0.51	0.47	0.44	0.41	0.39	0.37	0.35	0.33	0.31	0.30
10	1.66	1.48	1.33	1.21	1.11	1.02	0.95	0.88	0.83	0.78	0.74	0.70	0.66	0.63	0.60
15	2.50	2.22	2.00	1.81	1.66	1.53	1.42	1.33	1.25	1.17	1.11	1.05	1.00	0.95	0.90
20	3.33	2.96	2.66	2.42	2.22	2.05	1.90	1.77	1.66	1.56	1.48	1.40	1.33	1.27	1.21
25	4.16	3.70	3.33	3.03	2.77	2.56	2.38	2.22	2.08	1.96	1.85	1.75	1.66	1.58	1.51
30	5.00	4.44	4.00	3.63	3.33	3.07	2.85	2.66	2.50	2.35	2.22	2.10	2.00	1.90	1.81
35	5.83	5.18	4.66	4.24	3.88	3.59	3.33	3.11	2.91	2.74	2.59	2.45	2.33	2.22	2.12
40	6.66	5.92	5.33	4.84	4.44	4.10	3.81	3.55	3.33	3.13	2.96	2.80	2.66	2.54	2.42
45	7.50	6.66	6.00	5.45	5.00	4.61	4.28	4.00	3.75	3.52	3.33	3.15	3.00	2.85	2.72
50	8.33	7.40	6.66	6.06	5.55	5.12	4.76	4.44	4.16	3.92	3.70	3.50	3.33	3.17	3.03
55	9.16	8.14	7.33	6.66	6.11	5.64	5.23	4.88	4.58	4.31	4.07	3.86	3.66	3.49	3.33
60	10.00	8.88	8.00	7.27	6.66	6.15	5.71	5.33	5.00	4.70	4.44	4.21	4.00	3.81	3.63
65	10.83	9.63	8.66	7.87	7.22	6.66	6.19	5.77	5.41	5.09	4.81	4.56	4.33	4.12	3.93
70	11.66	10.37	9.33	8.48	7.77	7.17	6.66	6.22	5.83	5.49	5.18	4.91	4.66	4.44	4.24
75	12.50	11.11	10.00	9.09	8.33	7.69	7.14	6.66	6.25	5.88	5.55	5.26	5.00	4.76	4.54
80	13.33	11.85	10.66	9.69	8.88	8.20	7.61	7.11	6.66	6.27	5.92	5.61	5.33	5.07	4.84
85	14.16	12.59	11.33	10.30	9.44	8.71	8.09	7.55	7.08	6.66	6.29	5.96	5.66	5.39	5.15
90	15.00	13.33	12.00	10.90	10.00	9.23	8.57	8.00	7.50	7.05	6.66	6.31	6.00	5.71	5.45
95	15.83	14.07	12.66	11.51	10.55	9.74	9.04	8.44	7.91	7.45	7.03	6.66	6.33	6.03	5.75
100	16.66	14.81	13.33	12.12	11.11	10.25	9.52	8.88	8.33	7.84	7.40	7.01	6.66	6.34	6.06
105	17.50	15.55	14.00	12.72	11.66	10.76	10.00	9.33	8.75	8.23	7.77	7.36	7.00	6.66	6.36
110	18.33	16.29	14.66	13.33	12.22	11.28	10.47	9.77	9.16	8.62	8.14	7.71	7.33	6.98	6.66
115	19.16	17.03	15.33	13.93	12.77	11.79	10.95	10.22	9.58	9.02	8.51	8.07	7.66	7.30	6.97
120	20.00	17.77	16.00	14.54	13.33	12.30	11.42	10.66	10.00	9.41	8.88	8.42	8.00	7.61	7.27

Verapamil Hydrochloride

Pharmacology

Calcium channel blocking agent that inhibits influx of extracellular calcium through slow channels across myocardial and vascular smooth muscle cell membranes

No effect on serum calcium concentration

Dilates coronary and systemic arteries

Diminishes myocardial oxygen requirements by reducing systemic blood pressure and cardiac contractility. Cardiac output is usually preserved, although decreases may be seen in patients with advanced heart failure

Vaughan-Williams class IV antiarrhythmic agent that slows atrioventricular node conduction and prolongs its effective refractory period—often prolongs P-R interval on ECG

May depress sinoatrial node automaticity and atrial conduction times. No significant effects on accessory bypass tract or intraventricular conduction times

(continued below)

Administrative Guidelines

Administer via precision control device into large vein, if possible

Continuously monitor ECG and carefully follow blood pressure and vital signs

Correct any underlying hypovolemia, if possible, before use

Do not administer disopyramide within 48 hours before or 24 hours after IV verapamil use (synergistic adverse cardiac effects)

Continuous intravenous infusion is not recommended because safety and efficacy have not been established

Do not administer concomitantly with IV dantrolene because cardiovascular collapse may result or with oral flecainide (synergistic adverse effects on the heart)

Contraindicated in patients with known hypersensitivity, severe hypotension, second-degree or third-degree block in the absence of a functioning

(continued below)

Exhibits local anesthetic action of uncertain clinical significance

Indications

Conversion of reentrant paroxysmal supraventricular tachydysrhythmias (PSVT) to sinus rhythm, including PSVT associated with accessory bypass tracts

Control of ventricular response in atrial flutter or fibrillation in the ***absence*** of an accessory bypass tract

Unlabeled Uses. Coronary vasospasm, uncontrolled hypertension, hypertrophic cardiomyopathies, control and suppression of multifocal atrial tachycardia, refractory coronary vasospasm, hyperdynamic or hypertrophic syndromes associated with hypotension

artificial pacemaker, cardiogenic shock, advanced heart failure (unless secondary to supraventricular tachycardia), sick sinus syndrome (unless functioning artificial ventricular pacemaker in place), atrial fibrillation and flutter with an accessory bypass tract, ventricular tachycardia, and within several hours of intravenous beta-blocker therapy

Use with caution in patients with heart failure and severe ventricular dysfunction; idiopathic hypertrophic cardiomyopathy; supratentorial tumors (may increase intracranial pressure); preexcitation syndromes; Duchenne's muscular dystrophy (may precipitate respiratory failure) with hepatic or renal impairment; in those receiving highly protein bound drugs; and in the presence of oral quinidine, digitalis, or cyclosporine therapy

Overdosage may manifest by nausea, weakness, confusion, slurred speech, hypotension, and bradydysrhythmias. Manage with general supportive treatment and consider beta-agonists, intravenous calcium salts, vasopressors, temporary pacing, and other appropriate resuscitative measures. There is no documented role for dialysis in this setting

Verapamil Hydrochloride

Pharmacokinetics

Onset of Action. 1–2 minutes

Peak Effects. 5–15 minutes

Duration of Action. 30 minutes–6 hours

Plasma (Distribution) Half-Life. 4 minutes

Tissue (Elimination) Half-Life. 2–8 hours

Metabolism. Via the liver with 70% excreted in the kidney as inactive metabolites. Highly protein bound

Dosing Information

Initial Dose. 2.5–5.0 mg (0.038–0.075 mg/kg) slow IV push over 3 minutes. May repeat 2.5 to 10 mg (0.038–0.15 mg/kg) after 15 to 30 minutes if necessary

Maximum Dose. 20 mg (0.30 mg/kg) over 30 minutes

Severe Hepatic or Renal Dysfunction. 2.5–10 mg (0.038–0.15 mg/kg) initially. Do not repeat unless essential. Reduce second dose and wait 60–90 minutes before administration

How Supplied

2.5 mg/mL—2-mL ampuls and vials of 5 mg
4-mL ampuls and vials of 10 mg

Potential Drug Interaction

Potentiation of Verapamil Effects. Beta-blockers, disopyramide, warfarin, phenytoin, salicylates, sulfonamides, dantrolene, sulfonylureas, quinidine, cimetidine, antihypertensive medications, diuretics, vasodilators, angiotensin converting enzyme inhibitors, flecainide

Antagonism of Verapamil Effects. Rifampin, calcium or vitamin D, phenobarbital

Possibly Potentiated by Verapamil. Lithium, digoxin, cyclosporine, carbamazepine, dantrolene, inhalational anesthetics that depress the myocardium, neuromuscular blockers, metoprolol, methyldopa, prazosin, quinidine, theophylline

Verapamil Hydrochloride

Principal Adverse Effects

CNS. Headache, seizures, dizziness, fatigue, insomnia, mental depression, nystagmus

CV. Congestive heart failure, heart block, asystole, bradycardia, hypotension, syncope, pulmonary edema, ventricular tachydysrhythmias, chest pain

GI. Abdominal discomfort, nausea, dyspepsia, ileus

GU. Frequency, impotence, dysmenorrhea

Allergic. Rash, pruritus, urticaria, bronchospasm

Miscellaneous. Flushing, diaphoresis, arthralgia, gynecomastia, vasculitis, alopecia, blurred vision, Stevens-Johnson syndrome, erythema multiforme

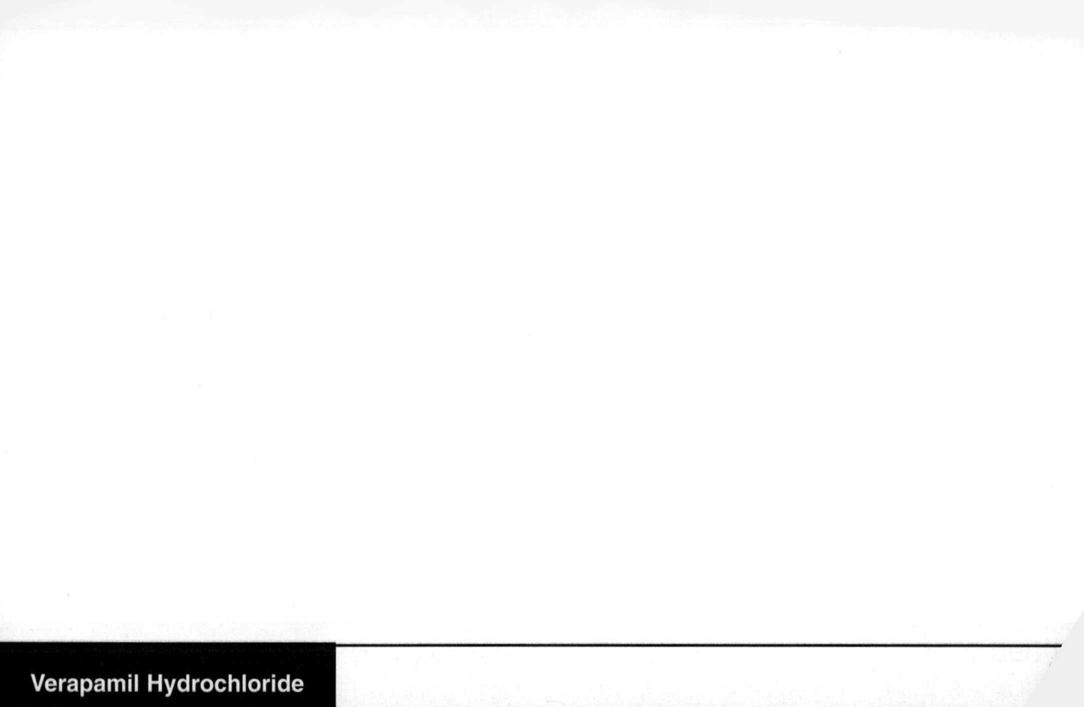

Verapamil Hydrochloride

Verapamil Hydrochloride

100 mg in 2

■ Infusion Rate in mL/hr (pump setting) ■ Drug Dose in mg/hr

mL/hr	mg/hr	mL/hr	mg/hr	mL/hr	mg/hr	mL/hr	mg/hr	mL/hr	mg/hr	mL/hr	mg/hr
1	0.4	21	8.4	41	16.4	61	24.4	81	32.4	101	40.4
2	0.8	22	8.8	42	16.8	62	24.8	82	32.8	102	40.8
3	1.2	23	9.2	43	17.2	63	25.2	83	33.2	103	41.2
4	1.6	24	9.6	44	17.6	64	25.6	84	33.6	104	41.6
5	2.0	25	10.0	45	18.0	65	26.0	85	34.0	105	42.0
6	2.4	26	10.4	46	18.4	66	26.4	86	34.4	106	42.4
7	2.8	27	10.8	47	18.8	67	26.8	87	34.8	107	42.8
8	3.2	28	11.2	48	19.2	68	27.2	88	35.2	108	43.2
9	3.6	29	11.6	49	19.6	69	27.6	89	35.6	109	43.6
10	4.0	30	12.0	50	20.0	70	28.0	90	36.0	110	44.0
11	4.4	31	12.4	51	20.4	71	28.4	91	36.4	111	44.4
12	4.8	32	12.8	52	20.8	72	28.8	92	36.8	112	44.8
13	5.2	33	13.2	53	21.2	73	29.2	93	37.2	113	45.2
14	5.6	34	13.6	54	21.6	74	29.6	94	37.6	114	45.6
15	6.0	35	14.0	55	22.0	75	30.0	95	38.0	115	46.0
16	6.4	36	14.4	56	22.4	76	30.4	96	38.4	116	46.4
17	6.8	37	14.8	57	22.8	77	30.8	97	38.8	117	46.8
18	7.2	38	15.2	58	23.2	78	31.2	98	39.2	118	47.2
19	7.6	39	15.6	59	23.6	79	31.6	99	39.6	119	47.6
20	8.0	40	16.0	60	24.0	80	32.0	100	40.0	120	48.0

DRUG DOSE in mg/kg/min

Patient's Weight kg / lbs	40 / 88	45 / 99	50 / 110	55 / 121	60 / 132	65 / 143	70 / 154	75 / 165	80 / 176	85 / 187	90 / 198	95 / 209	100 / 220	105 / 231	110 / 242
Infusion Rate in mL/hr															
5	0.05	0.04	0.04	0.04	0.03	0.03	0.03	0.03	0.03	0.02	0.02	0.02	0.02	0.02	0.02
10	0.10	0.09	0.08	0.07	0.07	0.06	0.06	0.05	0.05	0.05	0.04	0.04	0.04	0.04	0.04
15	0.15	0.13	0.12	0.11	0.10	0.09	0.09	0.08	0.08	0.07	0.07	0.06	0.06	0.06	0.05
20	0.20	0.18	0.16	0.15	0.13	0.12	0.11	0.11	0.10	0.09	0.09	0.08	0.08	0.08	0.07
25	0.25	0.22	0.20	0.18	0.17	0.15	0.14	0.13	0.13	0.12	0.11	0.11	0.10	0.10	0.09
30	0.30	0.27	0.24	0.22	0.20	0.18	0.17	0.16	0.15	0.14	0.13	0.13	0.12	0.11	0.11
35	0.35	0.31	0.28	0.25	0.23	0.22	0.20	0.19	0.17	0.16	0.16	0.15	0.14	0.13	0.13
40	0.40	0.36	0.32	0.29	0.27	0.25	0.23	0.21	0.20	0.19	0.18	0.17	0.16	0.15	0.15
45	0.45	0.40	0.36	0.33	0.30	0.28	0.26	0.24	0.22	0.21	0.20	0.19	0.18	0.17	0.16
50	0.50	0.44	0.40	0.36	0.33	0.31	0.29	0.27	0.25	0.24	0.22	0.21	0.20	0.19	0.18
55	0.55	0.49	0.44	0.40	0.37	0.34	0.31	0.29	0.28	0.26	0.24	0.23	0.22	0.21	0.20
60	0.60	0.53	0.48	0.44	0.40	0.37	0.34	0.32	0.30	0.28	0.27	0.25	0.24	0.23	0.22
65	0.65	0.58	0.52	0.47	0.43	0.40	0.37	0.35	0.32	0.31	0.29	0.27	0.26	0.25	0.24
70	0.70	0.62	0.56	0.51	0.47	0.43	0.40	0.37	0.35	0.33	0.31	0.29	0.28	0.27	0.25
75	0.75	0.67	0.60	0.55	0.50	0.46	0.43	0.40	0.38	0.35	0.33	0.32	0.30	0.29	0.27
80	0.80	0.71	0.64	0.58	0.53	0.49	0.46	0.43	0.40	0.38	0.36	0.34	0.32	0.30	0.29
85	0.85	0.76	0.68	0.62	0.57	0.52	0.49	0.45	0.43	0.40	0.38	0.36	0.34	0.32	0.31
90	0.90	0.80	0.72	0.65	0.60	0.55	0.51	0.48	0.45	0.42	0.40	0.38	0.36	0.34	0.33
95	0.95	0.84	0.76	0.69	0.63	0.58	0.54	0.51	0.47	0.45	0.42	0.40	0.38	0.36	0.35
100	1.00	0.89	0.80	0.73	0.67	0.62	0.57	0.53	0.50	0.47	0.44	0.42	0.40	0.38	0.36
105	1.05	0.93	0.84	0.76	0.70	0.65	0.60	0.56	0.52	0.49	0.47	0.44	0.42	0.40	0.38
110	1.10	0.98	0.88	0.80	0.73	0.68	0.63	0.59	0.55	0.52	0.49	0.46	0.44	0.42	0.40
115	1.15	1.02	0.92	0.84	0.77	0.71	0.66	0.61	0.57	0.54	0.51	0.48	0.46	0.44	0.42
120	1.20	1.07	0.96	0.87	0.80	0.74	0.69	0.64	0.60	0.56	0.53	0.51	0.48	0.46	0.44

Index

D

E

F

G

H

I

K